DIVERTICULITIS CC
THE ULTIMATE COOKBOOK WITH 300 RECIPES TO KEEP YOU HEALTHY

Table of Contents

Most people don't know the connection between diet and diverticulitis. Often, patients don't have a healthy diet because they assume that any food that is not severely processed will keep them from developing diverticulitis. However, consuming a proper dietary regime lowers your chances of developing this condition by as much as 50%.

Diverticulitis is a condition in which small pouches form in the tissues of the colon. These pouches are very painful and may increase your temp. if they become infected. The disease is a result of one or more of three main factors: history (genetic predisposition), personal habits, or previous infections acquired (acquired immunity).

Diverticulitis is a painful condition, which affects hundreds of thousands of people in the United States alone. This condition is most likely to occur during your senior years, but the earlier you treat it the less chance you have of experiencing significant health problems.

Diverticulitis is caused by the inflammation of the diverticula, which are small pouches in the wall of the colon. Diverticulosis is a condition in which these pouches are present without any symptoms. The exact cause of diverticulitis is not known. Risk factors include prolonged periods sitting on the toilet, straining during bowel movements, and a sedentary lifestyle. The risk increases with age and those who have had previous surgery on their abdomen are at particular risk.

Pain in your lower left abdomen is one of the symptoms that may occur after eating certain foods, particularly high-fiber foods such as nuts or seeds, corn or popcorn, and hard fruits such as apples or pears. Other symptoms include fever and constipation or diarrhea that lasts from several days to a few weeks. If you have these symptoms along with blood in your stool you may be diagnosed with diverticular bleeding, which requires urgent medical attention because it can lead to complications including peritonitis (inflammation of the abdominal cavity) and abscesses (pus-filled pockets).

Diverticular bleeding often occurs after straining during a bowel movement or after intense coughing fits brought on by an upper respiratory infection. Eating a high-fiber diet is another common cause of diverticular bleeding, and those who eat a lot of nuts and seeds may be more susceptible to this form of the condition. Diverticular bleeding may also occur after certain types of surgery on the abdomen, such as hernia repair, or after trauma to the abdomen.

Treatment for diverticular bleeding depends on its severity. Mild episodes usually resolve without treatment, but you may need to take stool softeners or laxatives to relieve constipation and prevent straining at the next bowel movement. You should also avoid hard or rough foods that can cause further damage if they become lodged in your colon.

The Diverticulitis Diet

The diverticulitis diet, or the diverticulosis diet, is designed to alleviate the symptoms of diverticulitis. It is also recommended for those who suffer from diverticular disease. The diet is meant to reduce pressure on the colon, which will prevent future flare-ups of diverticulitis. Although not a cure for diverticular disease, the diverticulitis diet can help reduce flare-ups and complications. The main recommendation for a diverticulitis diet is to eat low-fiber foods with lots of fluid intake. This helps decrease strain on your digestive system and prevents hard stools from being formed in your intestines. The type of foods that are high in fiber includes whole grains, wheat bran products, high-fiber cereals, and dried beans and peas. These foods should be avoided when you have a diverticular disease because they can cause inflammation of your intestinal walls and lead to complications such as obstruction or bleeding in your colon.

As always, consult a physician prior to making any changes to your eating habits

When you eat a diet that does not meet your requirements for nutrients and vitamins, toxins will build up in the digestive tract, leading to inflammation and symptoms of diverticulitis. Avoiding processed foods as much as possible will help you eliminate these toxins from your body. Lifestyle changes will also increase your chances of developing diverticulitis.

Avoid foods that have been over-processed as much as possible. You should avoid any foods with preservatives or artificial components in them. The more organic the food you eat, the better for your body.

Eat iron-rich foods. Your body also needs iron to produce red blood cells, which help deliver oxygen to your organs and tissues. Sources of natural iron include lean meats, fish, legumes, and green leafy vegetables. If you do not consume these types of food regularly you will be deficient in this important nutrient. When you are deficient in iron, the body absorbs calcium instead and diverticulitis may develop because of it.

Eat a lot of foods that are rich in vitamin C. Vitamin C enhances the body's immune defenses and lowers stomach acid production. It also prevents scurvy by providing the body with vitamin C, which is a water-soluble antioxidant. Foods that contain high amounts of vitamin C include citrus fruits, broccoli, brussels sprouts, and papaya.

Drink plenty of water. When your body is dehydrated it sends a signal to your colon to conserve water. In this situation, your colon doesn't release excess fluid into the intestines as it normally would and this can cause constipation.

Diverticular disease is one of the most common conditions in Western countries, with a particular presence in the United States, Europe, and Australia. According to a 2011 study by the US National Institutes of Health's National Library of Medicine (NIH/NLM), as many as 60 percent of Western people over the age of 70 have diverticular disease, and that number has only grown over the past decade. The disease encompasses three conditions: diverticulosis, diverticulitis, and diverticular bleeding. All of these involve the development of small sacs or pockets in the wall of the colon, called diverticula.

In a healthy individual, the colon is smooth and muscular, but those with diverticular disease have areas where the muscle has weakened (often due to age, because new cells don't rejuvenate as quickly as we get older)—the areas where diverticula are likely to form. From there, the condition can progress through two phases: diverticulosis and diverticulitis.

Diverticulosis

On its own, diverticulosis is not a source of concern—some live a healthy life with no symptoms at all. For others, diverticulosis may cause issues similar to irritable bowel syndrome (IBS), such as disruptive changes to regular bowel habits (including diarrhea, constipation, or fluctuation between the two). If stool gets trapped in the pouches (diverticula), it can cause diverticulosis to progress to diverticulitis. Approximately up to 15 to 20 percent of individuals with diverticulosis will see it turn into diverticulitis and this rate increases with age.

Diverticulitis

Diverticulitis happens when the diverticula become inflamed or infected. This can be an acute condition, meaning it's temporary and heals in a short amount of time, or chronic, meaning it's a long-term condition that may heal but never entirely goes away. Symptoms of diverticulitis may include diarrhea, abdominal pain (typically in the lower-left portion of the abdomen), cramping, constipation, fever, bleeding, and bloating. With diverticulitis, you may experience any combination of these symptoms.

The Progression

There are four stages of diverticulitis, which doctors measure using the Hinchey classification method. It's important to understand what stage you're in because if left untreated, diverticulitis can become a chronic issue, leading to bacterial infection or tears in the wall of your colon.

These are the different stages of the Hinchey Classification:

Stage 0: Mild Clinical Diverticulitis. Symptoms include pain in your lower left abdomen, fever, and elevated white blood cell count. In this stage, you are likely just beginning to experience symptoms and may not have confirmed your diverticulitis diagnosis through digital imagery or surgery.

Stage I: Pericolic Abscess or Phlegmon. The localized inflammation (which is causing the pain in your lower left abdomen) can lead to an abscess, or pocket, in the fat that surrounds the colon. If untreated, it can fill with pus and become infected.

Stage II: Pelvic, Intra-abdominal, or Retroperitoneal Abscess. The abscess has filled with pus or infected fluid, and you may be experiencing abdominal pain, constipation or diarrhea, fever, or vomiting.

Stage III: Generalized Purulent Peritonitis. The abscess is showing signs of bursting, which would drain pus into the abdomen and potentially lead to infection. This stage often requires surgery.

Stage IV: Generalized Fecal Peritonitis. At this stage, the abscess has burst and the fecal matter has released into the abdomen, a condition that can cause a dangerous infection, leading to sepsis and even death.

Individuals with uncomplicated diverticulitis (stages 0 to I) are usually able to manage the disease by following a high-fiber diet or, when in an active flare-up, with antibiotics and a clear liquid diet (also known as bowel rest). However, if you have substantial scarring or infected tissue, you may need to have that part of your colon surgically taken out to prevent the disease from getting worse.

Think of your colon like a balloon: it can only stretch so much prior to it pops. Recurring constipation or blockages will stretch your colon in much the same way. As you age, the strength of your colon decreases, which is why diverticulosis disproportionately affects those over the age of 70. The good news? A high-fiber diet can help prevent this added pressure on the colon.

Causes

Digestive disorders are notoriously challenging to narrow down to one cause, and thus doctors have not yet pinpointed a single source for diverticular disease. However, many factors may increase your chances of developing it, including a low-fiber diet, consuming red meat more than twice per week, certain medications, obesity, using tobacco products, lack of exercise, increased age, and genetics.

Low Fiber Intake. A low-fiber diet (including high red meat consumption) can lead to constipation, which makes it harder for you to pass stool and puts pressure on your colon. Researchers believe it is this pressure that weakens the bowel tissue and, over time, causes diverticula to form in the wall of the colon.

Medication. Some medications, like steroids and certain pain relievers, can increase your risk of developing diverticulitis. Nonsteroidal anti-inflammatory drugs (NSAIDs) such as aspirin and ibuprofen, in particular, can be very problematic. Consider these statistics from a 2011 NIH/NLM study: Of nearly a thousand people with diverticulitis, those who took aspirin more than twice per week were 25 percent more likely to experience complications than those who were not using NSAIDs. This is because NSAIDs have been proven to damage the lining of the intestinal tract.

Lifestyle Factors. Weight plays a significant role in your likelihood of developing diverticulitis, as excess fat stored in the abdominal cavity causes increased pressure on the colon and raises your risk of developing diverticula. Studies have shown that smokers are also at a higher risk of diverticular disease because smoking has been shown to raise your chances of perforations (tiny tears in the lining of the bowel that weaken the tissues). Finally, decreased or low movement (less than thirty mins of exercise per day) can lead to constipation, a huge contributor to diverticulitis development. Regular physical activity can help prevent diverticulitis by keeping food moving through your digestive tract.

Age. As you get older, the muscles in your colon weaken, increasing your likelihood of developing diverticular disease. In Western countries, it is estimated that 10 percent of people over age 40, and 50 percent of people over age 60, will be diagnosed with diverticulosis. That number keeps climbing the older you get.

Genetics. Unfortunately, sometimes your chances of developing diverticular disease live in your DNA, no matter your diet or lifestyle. Though there is no published study that has been able to identify a genetic link to diverticular disease, observational data does suggest the relationship, as there are differences in where the diverticula form depending on ethnicity. In Western countries, diverticula most commonly form in the descending parts of the colon, while in Asian countries, diverticula occur primarily in the ascending colon. These differences have led researchers to believe there could be genetic factors affecting the origin of diverticulitis.

In a study by Deniels and colleagues (2014), it is emphasized how important it is to manage diverticulosis to prevent diverticulitis. Diverticulitis has a high risk of recurrence (25%) and a non-negligible risk of surgery (17%). The authors of the study suggest that a high-fiber diet is a key to preventing diverticulitis and recommend a fiber intake of 20 gm/day. The conclusion is supported by other studies in which it was found that a high-fiber diet with more than 30 gm/day does not increase the risk of diverticulosis, it decreases the risk.

The recommendations made by Deniels and colleagues (2014) are supported by other studies such as those of Mozaffarian et al. (2004) who found that whole grains, fruit, and vegetables are associated with lower risks of diverticular disease, while processed meat is associated with increased risk. The authors conclude that an increase in fiber intake could have prevented up to one-fifth of diverticular disease cases.

In conclusion, a high-fiber diet may prevent diverticulosis and reduce the risk of developing complications such as diverticulitis or surgery.

Symptoms of Diverticulitis

Many diverticulitis patients do not experience daily symptoms outside of a flare. This, as you can imagine, makes diagnosis difficult outside of routine tests for general digestive issues. This isn't the reality for all patients: however, some experience warning signs or symptoms including:

Severe Constipation

Constipation can become so severe in diverticulitis patients that it prevents the passage of both gas and stool through the big intestine, and hence, a person is unable to pass the unwanted nitrogenous wastes out of the body.

Severe Pain in the Abdomen

Some may argue that abdominal pain is the most frequent symptom as over 95% of patients experience cramps in the left lower portion of the abdomen. These cramps can vary from person to person but have been generally described as an achy, dull, or even sharp pain in some cases. At times, this pain may radiate to the lower back. The pain is sudden and severe in most cases, but it can also be mild in some cases.

Fever

Many patients experience light fever in the early stages of diverticulitis and though it isn't a defining factor it does suggest the presence of an underlying infection. It is often associated with altered bowel habits, chills, or both.

Diverticular Bleeding

Though bleeding isn't common, it does occur in some patients. On the off chance that you have to bleed, it can be serious. Luckily, the bleeding in some cases may also stop on its own without requiring any form of treatment. Be that as it may, if you begin to experience any form of bleeding from your rectum, regardless of the amount, you should see a medical professional immediately.

To discover the site of the bleeding and stop it, a specialist may play out a colonoscopy. Your specialist may likewise utilize an automated tomography (CT) check or an angiogram to discover the bleeding site. An angiogram is a unique sort of x-beam in which your specialist strings a dainty, adaptable tube through an extensive corridor, frequently from your crotch to the bleeding region.

Urinary Symptoms

Another symptom that is not as widely linked to diverticulitis is urinary tract issues. These can vary from a burning sensation during urination, frequent urination, and other urinary-related issues due to the position of the bladder and colon in the body.

Nausea and Vomiting

Diverticulitis patients often suffer from indigestion-related symptoms such as nausea, vomiting, and heartburn.

Diverticulitis, when controlled, often doesn't severely affect your life outside of a flare. On the flip side, however, when the symptoms are left uncontrolled till it's too late, several more serious complications can pop up as a result. Including, but not limited to, intestinal perforation, fistula or abscess formation, peritonitis, bleeding, and stricture (blockade).

These complications, however, are often rare and mainly in patients who already have a compromised or weak immune system, for example, those with previous underlying autoimmune or chronic illnesses such as AIDs, cancer, heart disease, and also diabetes. Or some patients who have been taking steroids for a long period.

Benefits of a Diverticulitis Diet

Diet is one of the essential power tools we have to prevent and cure diverticulitis. A diet high in fiber will limit the number of toxins that accumulate in your colon, helping reduce or eliminate diverticulitis. In addition, a diet high in fruit and vegetables will provide you with essential nutrients your body needs to maintain healthy cells and tissues. Here are the benefits of following a diverticulitis diet:

- Helps reduce toxins and harmful bacteria in your colon
- Promotes proper digestion and elimination
- Controls blood sugar levels and cholesterol levels in your body
- Helps prevent heart disease, stroke, cancer, and diabetes

Diet and Diverticulitis

Diet may or may not play a role in diverticulitis, according to experts. There are no foods that all people with diverticulitis should avoid. However, you may discover that particular foods improve or aggravate your illness. If you have an intense case of diverticulitis, your doctor may advise you to cut back on your fiber consumption for a bit. For a few days, they may urge you to forgo solid foods entirely and stick to a clear liquid diet. This will also allow your digestive system to rest. Your doctor may advise you to eat more high-fiber meals when your symptoms improve. High-fiber diets have been associated with a lower risk of diverticulitis in some studies. Other studies have looked into the potential advantages of dietary or supplementary fiber for diverticular disease, although the role of fiber is still unknown. Limiting your intake of red meat, high-fat dairy items, and refined grain goods may also be recommended by your doctor. People who take a diet high in these items are more likely to develop diverticulitis than people who take a diet high in fruits, vegetables, and whole grains, according to big cohort research. Diet can help you manage diverticulitis and your digestive health in general.

Chapter 3. How to Diagnose Diverticulitis

Diverticulitis is often diagnosed via a normal X-ray or a colonoscopy, a test used to peer inside the rectum and whole colon to screen for colon malignancy or polyps or to assess the source of rectal death.

Because of the side effects and seriousness of the disease, a patient might be assessed and analyzed by an essential consideration doctor, a crisis division doctor, a specialist, or a gastroenterologist—a specialist who works in digestive diseases.

Blood Tests

A blood test includes drawing a patient's blood at the hospital and sending the example to a lab for examination. The blood test can demonstrate the nearness of irritation or paleness—a condition in which red platelets are less or littler than ordinary, which keeps the body's cells from getting enough oxygen.

Colonoscopy

The colonoscopy is performed at the hospital or an outpatient focus by a gastroenterologist. Before the test, the patient's social insurance supplier will give composed entrails prep directions to take after at home. The patient may need to take after an unmistakable fluid eating routine for 1 to 3 days prior to the test.

The individual may likewise need to take intestinal medicines and bowel purges the night prior to the test.

The patient will lie on a table while the gastroenterologist embeds an adaptable tube into the rear-end. A little camera on the tube sends a video picture of the intestinal coating to a PC screen. The test can demonstrate diverticulosis and diverticular sickness.

Examining Your Lower GI (Gastrointestinal) Arrangement

A lower GI arrangement is an X-ray exam that is utilized to take a gander at the digestive organ. The test is performed at a doctor's facility or an outpatient focus by an X-ray specialist, and the pictures are translated by a radiologist. Anesthesia is not required.

The doctor may give composed inside prep guidelines to take after at home prior to the test. The patient might be requested that take a reasonable fluid eating regimen for 1 to 3 days prior to the procedure. A diuretic or douche might be utilized prior to the test. A purgative is a pharmaceutical that extricates stool and expands solid discharges.

A bowel purge includes flushing water or purgative into the rectum utilizing a unique squirt bottle. These drugs cause the runs, so the patient ought to remain nearby to a restroom amid the inside prep. For the test, the patient will lie on a table while the radiologist embeds an adaptable tube into the individual's rear-end.

The colon is loaded with barium: making indications of diverticular illness appear entire more plainly on x beams. For a few days, hints of barium in the digestive organ can make stools white or light-hued. Douches and rehashed defecations may bring about butt-centric soreness. A doctor will give specific directions about eating and drinking after the test.

CT Scans (Mechanized Tomography)

A CT sweep of the colon is the most widely recognized test used to analyze Diverticular infection. CT filters utilize a mix of x beams and PC innovation to make three-dimensional (3-D) pictures. For a CT sweep, the individual might be given a beverage and an infusion of exceptional color called contrast medium. CT checks require the individual to lie on a table that slides into a passage molded gadget where the x beams are taken.

The technique is performed in an outpatient focus or a doctor's facility by an x-beam expert, and the pictures are deciphered by a radiologist. Anesthesia is not required. CT sweeps can distinguish diverticulosis and affirm its analysis.

Chapter 4. The 3 Stages of Diverticulitis

The Diet Stages

There are three main stages to the diverticulitis diet: managing an active flare-up, recovering from it, and preventing it in the future. Throughout each step, you must listen to your body and make diet adjustments slowly, adding one or two new foods at a time while closely monitoring your symptoms.

During a Flare-Up: Clear Fluids

If your flare-up symptoms are extreme, you may need to give your bowel a period of rest. A clear fluid diet will help your body recuperate because it may be temporarily unable to tolerate any solid foods. Take note that this is not meant to be a long-term diet—you should follow it for only a couple of days. Restricting yourself to a clear fluid diet for any length of time may cause you to feel weak, light-headed, exhausted, and hungry. Other symptoms include excessive weight loss, muscle wasting, and depletion of vitamins and minerals. These symptoms occur because it's challenging to meet the body's daily caloric requirements for protein, carbohydrates, and fat through a clear fluid diet. To provide your body with enough energy, you need to consume almost 200 grams of carbohydrates throughout the day. If you have blood sugar challenges such as low blood sugar or diabetes, you may want to monitor your blood sugars during this stage.

After a Flare-Up: Low-Residue Foods

A low-residue (or low-fiber) diet acts as the reintroduction phase, after your flare-up symptoms have mostly passed but prior to your body is ready for high-fiber foods. "Residue" is the indigestible fiber that passes through the big intestine and then is excreted as a stool. This diet aims to reduce the number of bowel movements you have, which will, in turn, decrease the pain associated with the flare-up. Like the precise fluid stage, the low-residue diet is not meant to be a long-term lifestyle. You should

only follow it while you are recovering from inflammation and flare-up pain. Once the pain subsides, you can start introducing more high-fiber foods, working your way up to a high-fiber diet.

Flare-Up Prevention: High-Fiber Foods

This final stage of the diverticulitis diet is the maintenance and prevention phase—in other words, your regular eating routine. When you're not suffering or recovering from a flare-up, a high-fiber diet can protect against the development of diverticula by keeping bowel movements stable and accessible. However, you do not want to go from a low-fiber diet straight to a high-fiber diet, as this can damage your colon. Slow and steady is the rule when it comes to fiber increase: aim to increase your fiber intake by 2 to 4 grams per week till you reach the recommended amount for your age and biology. Keep in mind that as you increase your fiber.

What to Eat and Not to Eat During Each Stage of Diverticulitis

Diverticulosis can lead to three different stages of diverticulitis. In each stage, the symptoms are various, and depending on which stage an individual is in, they may have an additional chance of survival. Individuals at the early stages of diverticulosis usually do not experience any significant symptoms and can control the disease themselves with some minor lifestyle changes. Most people who endure this disease do not need medication or antibiotics and will heal within a few days or months with simple diet changes and exercise habits.

Stage 1

At the initial stages of diverticulitis, the ones that are caused by eating a diet high in fat and low in fiber will be treated with simple diet changes. Individuals at the early stages of developing diverticulosis should limit their consumption of red meat and other foods that are high in fat and processed foods containing preservatives or chemicals. Eating a fiber-rich diet is essential to prevent further inflammation and symptoms that can eventually lead to more severe stages. These groups of foods should consist of fruit, whole grains, and low-fat dairy products.

Stage 2

At the second stage of diverticulosis, foods high in fat content are still avoided, but a fiber-rich diet remains vital to prevent further inflammation. A diet that consists of foods like whole grains, fruits, and vegetables is crucial at this stage. A mixture of these foods with some lean meat can also be great for any bacteria present in one's colon. Many people will try to make a much healthier diet by consuming plenty of fiber and water.

Stage 3

At the final stage, all foods eaten should consist of fiber, and lean meat is not recommended to be consumed in big amounts. A low-fat diet is best followed with the goal being to reduce the inflammation from diverticulitis. Consuming foods like barley, pine nuts, flax seeds, wheat bran, and oat bran is a great way to get fiber. Because of the amount of fiber present in these foods, most people will crave sweets.

The leading cause of diverticulitis is the result of a diet that does not consist of enough fiber. Individuals who do not consume enough fiber are at high risk of developing diverticulitis. A diet rich in red meat, a variety of processed foods, and low fiber will increase one's chance of developing this disease. Those who have a family history or have had diverticulosis previously should also be mindful of their diet and incorporate more fiber into it.

Chapter 5. Shopping List

Fruits

- Apple Sauce
- Apples
- Apricots
- Bananas
- Dates

- Mangoes
- Oranges
- Peaches
- Prunes

- Apple Juice
- Lemon Juice
- Lime Juice

Juices

- Orange Juice
- Cranberry Juice

Vegetables

- Alfalfa Sprouts
- Artichoke Hearts
- Asparagus
- Avocados
- Black Olives
- Broccoli
- Butternut Squash
- Cabbage
- Carrots
- Cauliflower
- Celery
- Eggplants
- Garlic
- Green Bell Peppers (seedless)
- Green Olives
- Green Onions
- Leeks

- Mushrooms
- Lettuce
- Olives
- Onions
- Peas (frozen, cooked)
- Pimento
- Red Bell Peppers (seedless)
- Russet Potatoes
- Shallots
- Spinach
- Sugar Snap Peas
- Summer Squash
- Yellow Peppers (seedless)
- Tomatoes (seedless)
- Water chestnuts
- Zucchini
- Sweet Yams

Beans & Peas

- Black Beans
- Butter Beans
- Cannellini Beans
- Garbanzo Beans
- Canned Kidney Beans

- Lentils
- Canned Lima Beans
- Canned Navy Beans
- Canned Red Beans

Grains, Types of Bread & Other Starches

- All-Bran Cereal
- Barley
- Brown Rice
- Fiber One Cereal
- Long Grain Rice
- Oat Bran
- Rolled Oats

- Whole Wheat Tortellini
- Whole Wheat Flour
- Whole Wheat Pasta
- Whole Wheat Pita
- Whole Wheat Tortillas
- Whole Wheat Bread

Meats

- Crab Meat, Cooked
- Ground Chicken, Lean
- Ground Turkey, Lean
- Lean Ham

- Shrimp, big, skinned
- Canned Tuna Fish, in water
- Turkey Breast
- Chicken Breast

Dairy

- Cheddar Cheese (low fat)
- Cottage Cheese (low fat)
- Cream Cheese (low fat)
- Feta Cheese
- Monterrey Jack Cheese (low fat)

- Parmesan Cheese
- Eggs
- Half and half cream
- Milk, low fat
- Yogurt, low fat

Spices, Herbs & Oils

- Baking Powder
- Basil (fresh or dried)
- Canola Oil
- Cilantro (fresh)
- Cinnamon powder
- Cumin
- Curry Powder
- Dill, (fresh or dried)
- Italian Seasoning

- Nutmeg
- Olive Oil
- Oregano, (fresh and dried)
- Parsley, Italian (fresh)
- Sage (fresh)
- Tarragon (fresh)
- Thyme (fresh and dried)
- Vanilla

Condiments

- Vegetable Stock
- Chicken Stock
- Coconut Milk
- Dijon Mustard
- Honey
- Light Ranch Dressing
- Maple Syrup
- Mayonnaise, low fat
- Red Wine Vinegar

- Rice Vinegar
- Soy Sauce
- Sweet Pickle Relish
- Tarragon Vinegar
- Tomato Paste
- Tomato Sauce
- Tomato Puree
- Canned Tomato, cubed, seedless

Chapter 6. 90 Days Meal Plan

Days	Breakfast	Lunch	Snacks	Dinner
1	citrus sports drink	banana oat shake	mango pudding (dairy-free!) recipe	chicken bone broth
2	homemade orange gelatin	banana-apple smoothie	Banana oatmeal chocolate chip cookies (healthy!)	homemade beef stock
3	raspberry lemonade ice pops	Berrylicious smoothie	Larabar snack bar	three-ingredient sugar-free gelatin
4	homemade no pulp orange juice	buttermilk herb ranch dressing	kulfi Indian ice cream	cranberry-kombucha Jell-O
5	apple orange juice	citrus relish	easy no-bake key lime pie recipe	strawberry gummies
6	pineapple mint juice	chickpea pancakes recipe	Lemon cheesecake recipe (limoncello cake!)	fruity Jell-O stars
7	celery apple juice	red wine sangria recipe	French toast	sugar-free cinnamon jelly
8	homemade banana apple juice	salty dog cocktail recipe	dark chocolate with pomegranate seeds	homey clear chicken broth
9	sweet detox juice	simple syrup	covered bananas	oxtail bone broth
10	pineapple ginger juice	rose sangria recipe	hummus with tahini and turmeric	chicken bone broth with ginger and lemon
11	carrot orange juice	champagne holiday punch recipe	pineapple orange Creamsicle	vegetable stock
12	strawberry apple juice	white sangria	easy peach cobbler recipe with Bisquick	chicken vegetable soup
13	autumn energizer juice	raspberry mojitos with basil	healthy five-min strawberry pineapple sherbet	carrot ginger soup
14	Asian inspired wonton broth	margarita recipe	Best coconut milk ice cream (dairy-free!)	turkey sweet potato hash
15	mushroom, cauliflower, and cabbage broth	pink grapefruit margarita	lemon crinkle cookies recipe	chicken tenders with honey mustard sauce
16	Indian inspired vegetable stock	grapefruit basil sorbet	the best no-bake chocolate lasagna	chicken breasts with cabbage and mushrooms
17	beef bone broth	Bruleed grapefruit (Pamplemousse Brûlé)	easiest healthy watermelon smoothie recipe	duck with bok choy
18	ginger, mushroom, and cauliflower broth	frozen beeritas recipe	watermelon	beef with mushroom and broccoli
19	fish broth	spicy pineapple habanero margaritas	best orange Julius	beef with zucchini noodles
20	clear pumpkin broth	cranberry pomegranate margarita with spiced rim	mango pudding (dairy-free!) recipe	spiced ground beef

21	pork stock	Peach milkshake (copycat chik-fil-a peach shake recipe!)	Banana oatmeal chocolate chip cookies (healthy!)	ground beef with veggies
22	slow-cooker pork bone broth	jugo verde (green juice)	Larabar snack bar	ground beef with greens and tomatoes
23	strawberry overnight oats	perfect Manhattan recipe	kulfi Indian ice cream	chicken bone broth
24	ginger peach smoothie	frozen coconut mojito	easy no-bake key lime pie recipe	homemade beef stock
25	strawberry banana peanut butter smoothie	mulled lemonade recipe	Lemon cheesecake recipe (limoncello cake!)	three-ingredient sugar-free gelatin
26	granola	cucumber rose aperol spritz	French toast	cranberry-kombucha Jell-O
27	persimmon smoothie	pink grapefruit margarita	dark chocolate with pomegranate seeds	strawberry gummies
28	cranberry smoothie	strawberry margarita recipe	covered bananas	fruity Jell-O stars
29	kale apple smoothie	large-batch goombay smash Caribbean cocktails	hummus with tahini and turmeric	sugar-free cinnamon jelly
30	glowing skin smoothie	healthy vegan brownies	pineapple orange Creamsicle	homey clear chicken broth
31	cranberry sauce	green chicken soup	papaya-mango smoothie	Italian styled stuffed zucchini boats
32	chocolate tahini pumpkin smoothie	green risotto recipe	cantaloupe smoothie	chicken cutlets
33	spinach frittata	barbecue beef stir-fry	cantaloupe-mix smoothie	slow cooker salsa turkey
34	banana and pear pita pockets	chicken saffron rice pilaf	applesauce-avocado smoothie	sriracha lime chicken and apple salad
35	pear pancakes	stir-fry ground chicken and green beans	Pina colada smoothie	pan-seared scallops with lemon-ginger vinaigrette
36	ripe plantain bran muffins	stewed lamb	diced fruits	roasted salmon and asparagus
37	easy breakfast bran muffins	pulled chicken salad	avocado dip	orange and maple-glazed salmon
38	apple oatmeal	lemongrass beef	homemade hummus	cod with ginger and black beans
39	breakfast burrito wrap	beetroot carrot salad	almond butter sandwich	halibut curry
40	zucchini omelet	crunchy maple sweet potatoes	gluten-free muffins	chicken cacciatore
41	coconut chia seed pudding	veggie bowl	papaya-mango smoothie	chicken and bell pepper saute
42	spiced oatmeal	pomegranate salad	cantaloupe smoothie	chicken salad sandwiches

43	breakfast cereal	Dijon orange summer salad	cantaloupe-mix smoothie	rosemary chicken
44	sweet potato hash with sausage and spinach	pulao rice prawns	applesauce-avocado smoothie	gingered turkey meatballs
45	Cajun omelet	white radish crunch salad	Pina colada smoothie	turkey and kale saute
46	strawberry cashew chia pudding	apple and mushroom soup	diced fruits	turkey with bell peppers and rosemary
47	peanut butter banana oatmeal	spring watercress soup	avocado dip	mustard and rosemary pork tenderloin
48	overnight peach oatmeal	oyster sauce tofu	homemade hummus	thin-cut pork chops with mustardy kale
49	Mediterranean salmon and potato salad	potato and rosemary risotto	almond butter sandwich	beef tenderloin with savory blueberry sauce
50	celery soup	cheesy baked tortillas	gluten-free muffins	ground beef chili with tomatoes
51	pea tuna salad	smoky rice	papaya-mango smoothie	fish taco salad with strawberry avocado salsa
52	vegetable soup	zucchini lasagna	cantaloupe smoothie	beef and bell pepper stir-fry
53	carrot and turkey soup	greek chicken skewers	cantaloupe-mix smoothie	veggie pizza with cauliflower-yam crust
54	creamy pumpkin soup	roast beef	applesauce-avocado smoothie	toasted pecan quinoa burgers
55	chicken pea soup	banana cake	Pina colada smoothie	sizzling salmon and quinoa
56	coconut pancakes	grilled fish steaks	diced fruits	Italian styled stuffed zucchini boats
57	spinach frittata	apple pudding	avocado dip	chicken cutlets
58	banana and pear pita pockets	lamb chops	homemade hummus	slow cooker salsa turkey
59	pear pancakes	eggplant croquettes	almond butter sandwich	sriracha lime chicken and apple salad
60	ripe plantain bran muffins	cucumber egg salad	gluten-free muffins	pan-seared scallops with lemon-ginger vinaigrette
61	mango ginger smoothie	high-fiber dumplings	banana-bread muffins	grilled pear cheddar pockets
62	banana cacao smoothie	pizza made with bamboo fibers	berry fruit leathers	chicken and apple kale wraps
63	spinach and egg scramble with raspberries	vegetarian hamburgers	chocolate-covered banana slices	cauliflower rice pilaf
64	blackberry smoothie	pork steaks with avocado	coconut macaroons	fresh herb and lemon bulgur pilaf
65	veggie frittata	chicken with asparagus salad	banana ice cream	corn chowder
66	chocolate banana protein smoothie	hot pepper and lamb salmon	berry berry sorbet	strawberry and rhubarb soup

67	cocoa almond French toast	pork rolls à la ratatouille	oatmeal semisweet chocolate-chip cookies	chicken sandwiches
68	muesli with raspberries	pepper fillet with leek	coconut-lemon bars	tex-mex bean tostadas
69	mocha overnight oats	lamb chops with beans	flourless chocolate cake with berry sauce	fish tacos
70	baked banana-nut oatmeal cups	fillet of beef on spring vegetables	baked parsnip chips	cucumber almond gazpacho
71	pineapple green smoothie	Bolognese with zucchini noodles	lemon ricotta cake (crepe cake recipe)	pea and spinach carbonara
72	pumpkin bread	chicken with chickpeas	sweet fried plantains	sautéed broccoli with peanut sauce
73	banana-bran muffins	ham with chicory	French chocolate silk pie recipe	edamame lettuce wraps burgers
74	banana bread	pork medallions with asparagus and coconut curry	peanut butter oatmeal chocolate chip cookies (monster cookie recipe)	pizza stuffed spaghetti squash
75	chocolate-raspberry oatmeal	lamb with carrot and brussels sprouts spaghetti	banana-bread muffins	spinach and artichoke dip pasta
76	chai chia pudding	cabbage wrap	berry fruit leathers	grilled eggplant
77	apple cinnamon oatmeal	veal with asparagus	chocolate-covered banana slices	stuffed potatoes with salsa and beans
78	apple butter bran muffins	salmon with sesame seeds and mushrooms	coconut macaroons	mushroom quinoa veggie burgers
79	pineapple raspberry parfaits	stuffed trout with mushrooms	banana ice cream	turkey meatballs
80	berry chia pudding	salmon with basil and avocado	berry sorbet	sweet potato soup
81	spinach avocado smoothie	leek quiche with olives	oatmeal semisweet chocolate-chip cookies	minestrone soup
82	strawberry pineapple smoothie	fried egg on onions with sage	coconut-lemon bars	lentil soup
83	peach blueberry parfaits	quinoa mushroom risotto	flourless chocolate cake with berry sauce	grilled corn salad
84	raspberry yogurt cereal bowl	vegetarian lentil stew	baked parsnip chips	kale soup
85	avocado toast	lemon chicken soup with beans	lemon ricotta cake (crepe cake recipe)	pasta Faggioli
86	loaded pita pockets	high-fiber dumplings	sweet fried plantains	sweet potato gnocchi
87	pear pancakes	pizza made with bamboo fibers	French chocolate silk pie recipe	bean and ham soup
88	almond pancakes	vegetarian hamburgers	peanut butter oatmeal chocolate chip cookies (monster cookie recipe)	grilled pear cheddar pockets
89	avocado pancakes	pork steaks with avocado	banana-bread muffins	chicken and apple kale wraps
90	strawberry pancakes	chicken with asparagus salad	berry fruit leathers	cauliflower rice pilaf

Breakfast

1. Citrus Sports Drink

Preparation Time: five mins

Cooking Time: zero mins

Servings: eight

Ingredients:

- four teacups coconut water
- four big oranges juice (about one and half teacups), strained
- two tbsps lemon juice, strained
- two tbsps honey or maple syrup
- one tsp sea salt

Directions:

1. Place the coconut water, orange juice, lemon juice, honey, and salt in a jug or pitcher.
2. Stir till the salt is melted.
3. Serve cold.

Nutrition: Calories: 59; Fat: 1 gm; Carbs: 14 gm; Fiber: 1 gm; Protein: 1 gm; Sodium: 304 mg

2. Homemade Orange Gelatin

Preparation Time: four hrs and ten mins

Cooking Time: three mins

Servings: four

Ingredients:

- eight big juiced oranges (about three teacups), strained and divided
- two tbsps unflavored gelatin
- two tbsps honey or maple syrup

Directions:

1. Inside a big container, pour in half teacup of orange juice and sprinkle the gelatin. Whisk well and let it sit till the gelatin begins to set but is not quite smooth.
2. Inside a saucepot at low temp., pour in the rest of the two and half teacups of orange juice and cook till prior to boiling, for two-three mins.
3. Take out from the heat and pour the hot juice into the gelatin mixture. Include the honey or maple syrup; stir till the gelatin is melted.
4. Pour into an 8 x 8 inches baking dish and transfer to the fridge.
5. Cool for four hrs to set. Serve cold.

Nutrition: Calories: 127; Fat: 1 gm; Carbs: 28 gm; Fiber: 1 gm; Protein: 6 gm; Sodium: 2 mg

3. Raspberry Lemonade Ice Pops

Preparation Time: four hrs and ten mins

Cooking Time: zero mins

Servings: four ice pops

Ingredients:

- three teacups frozen raspberries
- one tsp lemon juice, strained
- quarter teacup coconut water
- quarter teacup honey or maple syrup

Directions:

1. Inside a mixer, puree the raspberries, lemon juice, and coconut water till smooth.
2. Pass the mixture through a fine-mesh strainer into a container, to take out the seeds. Stir in the honey till well mixed.
3. Divide the mixture equally among four popsicle molds and freeze till solid, for three-four hrs.

Nutrition: Calories: 120; Fat: 0 gm; Carbs: 31 gm; Fiber: 7 gm; Protein: 2 gm; Sodium: 2 mg

4. Homemade No Pulp Orange Juice

Preparation Time: five mins

Cooking Time: zero mins

Servings: one and half teacups

Ingredients:

- four oranges

Directions:

1. Lightly, squeeze the oranges on a hard surface to soften the exterior. Slice each orange in half.
2. Squeeze each orange over a fine-mesh strainer.
3. Gently, press the pulp to extract the liquid.
4. Serve over ice. Relish!

Nutrition: Calories: 50; Fat: 0.2 gm; Carbs: 11.5 gm; Protein: 0.8 gm

5. Apple Orange Juice

Preparation Time: five mins

Cooking Time: zero mins

Servings: two

Ingredients:

- one Gala apple, skinned, cored, and sliced
- 2 oranges, skinned, halved, and seeded
- two tsps honey (optional)
- three-quarter teacup water

Directions:

1. Squeeze each orange over a fine-mesh strainer.
2. Gently, press the pulp to extract as much liquid as possible.
3. Include in the apple, water, and orange juice in your blender and pulse.
4. Set a fine-mesh strainer inside a container prior to transferring your juice into the strainer.

5. Once again, gently press the pulp to take out all the liquid; then, discard it.
6. Stir in your honey; then serve over ice.

Nutrition: Calories: 180; Fat: 1 gm; Carbs: 43 gm; Fiber: 1 gm; Protein: 2 gm

6. Pineapple Mint Juice

Preparation Time: five mins.

Cooking Time: zero mins

Servings: four

Ingredients:

- three teacups pineapple, cored, sliced, and chunks
- 10-12 mint leaves, or as required
- two tbsps sugar, or as required (optional)
- one and half teacups water
- one teacup ice cubes

Directions:

1. Set the entire components into your blender, and pulse.
2. Set a fine-mesh strainer inside a container prior to transferring your juice into the strainer.
3. Gently, press the pulp to extract the liquid; then, discard it.
4. Serve over ice.
5. Relish!

Nutrition: Calories: 78; Fat: 1 gm; Carbs: 22 gm; Fiber: 2 gm; Protein: 1 gm

7. Celery Apple Juice

Preparation Time: five mins

Cooking Time: zero mins

Servings: two

Ingredients:

- twelve celery stalks, skinned and severed
- 3 apples, skinned, cored, seeded, and sliced
- one inch ginger root, skinned and severed
- 1/4 lemon juice
- two teacups water

Directions:

1. Set the entire components into your blender, and pulse.
2. Set a fine-mesh strainer inside a container prior to transferring your juice into the strainer.
3. Gently, press the pulp to extract the liquid; then, discard it.
4. Serve over ice.
5. Relish!

Nutrition: Calories: 119; Fat: 1 gm; Carbs: 29 gm; Fiber: 7 gm; Protein: 2 gm

8. Homemade Banana Apple Juice

Preparation Time: ten mins

Cooking Time: zero mins

Servings: two

Ingredients:

- 2 bananas, skinned and sliced
- 1/2 apple, skinned, cored, and severed
- one tbsp honey
- one and half teacups water

Directions:

1. Set the entire components into your blender, and pulse.
2. Set a fine-mesh strainer inside a container prior to transferring your juice into the strainer.
3. Gently, press the pulp to extract the liquid; then, discard it.
4. Serve over ice.
5. Relish!

Nutrition: Calories: 132; Fat: 2 gm; Carbs: 27 gm; Fiber: 3 gm; Protein: 4 gm

9. Sweet Detox Juice

Preparation Time: ten mins

Cooking Time: zero mins

Servings: two

Ingredients:

- two teacups baby spinach, severed
- 1 handful parsley, severed
- 1 green apple, skinned, cored, seeded, and sliced
- one big English cucumber, seeded and severed
- one inch ginger, skinned
- 1 lemon, juiced

Directions:

1. Set the entire components into your blender, and pulse.
2. Set a fine-mesh strainer inside a container prior to transferring your juice into the strainer.
3. Gently, press the pulp to extract the liquid; then, discard it.
4. Serve over ice.
5. Relish!

Nutrition: Calories: 209; Fat: 2 gm; Carbs: 48 gm; Fiber: 17 gm; Protein: 12 gm

10. Pineapple Ginger Juice

Preparation Time: thirty-five mins

Cooking Time: zero mins

Servings: seven teacups

Ingredients:

- 10 cups pineapple, severed
- 6 teacups water
- 3 Fuji apples, severed
- 4-inch ginger root, skinned and severed
- quarter teacup lemon juice

- quarter teacup sugar

Directions:

1. Set the entire components into your blender, and pulse.
2. Set a fine-mesh strainer inside a container prior to transferring your juice into the strainer.
3. Gently, press the pulp to extract the liquid; then, discard it.
4. Serve over ice.
5. Relish!

Nutrition: Calories: 71; Fat: 1 gm; Carbs: 20 gm; Fiber: 3 gm; Protein: 1 gm

11. **Carrot Orange Juice**

Preparation Time: fifteen mins

Cooking Time: zero mins

Servings: two

Ingredients:

- one medium yellow tomato, cut into wedges
- 1 orange, skinned and quartered
- 1 apple, skinned, cored, and severed
- 4 jumbo carrots, skinned and severed
- two teacups water

Directions:

1. Set the entire components into your blender, and pulse.
2. Set a fine-mesh strainer inside a container prior to transferring your juice into the strainer.
3. Gently, press the pulp to extract the liquid; then, discard it.
4. Serve over ice.
5. Relish!

Nutrition: Calories: 111; Fat: 1 gm; Carbs: 24 gm; Fiber: 1 gm; Protein: 2 gm

12. **Strawberry Apple Juice**

Preparation Time: five mins

Cooking Time: zero mins

Servings: eight-ten oz.

Ingredients:

- two teacups strawberries (tops taken out)
- one red apple, skinned, sowed, cored, and sliced
- one tbsp chia seeds
- one teacup water

Directions:

1. Set the entire components into your blender and pulse.
2. Set a fine-mesh strainer inside a container prior to transferring your juice into the strainer.
3. Gently, press the pulp to extract the liquid; then, discard it.

4. Include in your chia seeds. Then, leave to sit for almost five mins.
5. Serve over ice.
6. Relish!

Nutrition: Calories: 245; Fat: 5 gm; Carbs: 52 gm; Fiber: 7 gm; Protein: 4 gm

13. **Autumn Energizer Juice**

Preparation Time: ten mins

Cooking Time: zero mins

Servings: two

Ingredients:

- 2 pears, skinned, seeded, and severed
- 2 Ambrosia apples, skinned, cored, and severed
- 2 Granny Smith apples, skinned, cored, severed
- 2 mandarins, juiced
- two teacups sweet potato, skinned and severed
- 1-pint cape gooseberries
- 2-in ginger root, skinned

Directions:

1. Set the entire components into your blender, and pulse.
2. Set a fine-mesh strainer inside a container prior to transferring your juice into the strainer.
3. Gently, press the pulp to extract the liquid; then, discard it.
4. Serve over ice.
5. Relish!

Nutrition: Calories: 170; Fat: 3 gm; Carbs: 33 gm; Fiber: 9 gm; Protein: 4 gm

14. **Asian Inspired Wonton Broth**

Preparation Time: five mins

Cooking Time: one hr and thirty mins

Servings: two

Ingredients:

- one chicken thigh, skin on
- 1 carrot, coarsely severed
- one celery stalk, coarsely severed
- 1 small onion, quartered
- 3 dime-sized ginger pieces
- two tbsps Kosher salt
- quarter tsp turmeric
- one-eighth tsp MSG (don't leave it out)
- 5 white peppercorns (can be substituted with black)
- 1-liter water

Directions:

1. Transfer the entire components to your stockpot. Top with sufficient water to cover; then, allow slowly come to a boil, on high heat.

2. Switch to low heat. Simmer for almost one hr and thirty mins.
3. Set and pour the mixture through a fine-mesh strainer into a big container.
4. Taste and season with salt.
5. Serve warm.

Nutrition: Calories: 181; Fat: 7 gm; Carbs: 14 gm; Fiber: 1 gm; Protein: 14 gm

15. Mushroom, Cauliflower, and Cabbage Broth

Preparation Time: ten mins

Cooking Time: fifty mins

Servings: two

Ingredients:

- one big yellow onion
- one teacup celery stalks, severed
- 2 carrots, cubed or cubed
- 10 French beans
- 1/2 cabbage, cubed
- 1-2 stalks celery leaves
- one and half teacups mushrooms, sliced
- 8 florets cauliflower
- one tsp garlic, severed
- one tsp ginger, severed
- one tbsp oil
- 1 scallion stalk
- half tsp pepper, crushed

Directions:

1. Transfer the entire components to your stockpot. Top with sufficient water to cover; then, allow slowly come to a boil on high heat.
2. Switch to low heat. Simmer for fifty mins.
3. Set and pour the mixture through a fine-mesh strainer into a big container. Mash the vegetables well to extract all their juices.
4. Taste and season with salt.
5. Relish.

Nutrition: Calories: 141; Fat: 5 gm; Carbs: 22 gm; Fiber: 7 gm; Protein: 5 gm

16. Indian Inspired Vegetable Stock

Preparation Time: ten mins

Cooking Time: eleven mins

Servings: three

Ingredients:

- three-quarter teacup onions, roughly severed
- three-quarter teacup carrot, roughly severed
- three-quarter teacup tomatoes, roughly severed
- three-quarter teacup potatoes, roughly severed
- one tsp turmeric

- Salt, as required

Directions:

1. Transfer the entire components to your stockpot. Top with sufficient water to cover. Then, allow slowly come to a boil on high heat.
2. Switch to low heat. Simmer for eleven mins.
3. Set and pour the mixture through a fine-mesh strainer into a big container. Taste and season with salt.
4. Serve warm.
5. Relish!

Nutrition: Calories: 103; Fat: 0.2mg; Carbs: 23.3 gm; Fiber: 3.1 gm; Protein: 2.2 gm

17. Beef Bone Broth

Preparation Time: ten mins

Cooking Time: twelve hrs

Servings: eight

Ingredients:

- two lbs. beef bones
- 1 onion, severed in quarters
- two celery stalks, severed in half
- 2 carrots, severed in half
- 3 whole garlic pieces
- two bay leaves
- one tbsp salt
- Filtered water (enough to cover bones)

Directions:

1. Transfer the bones and vegetables to your stockpot. Top with sufficient water to cover. Then, allow slowly come to a boil on high heat.
2. Switch to low heat. Simmer for almost two hrs and up to twelve hrs.
3. Set and pour the mixture through a fine-mesh strainer into a big container. Taste and season with salt.
4. Serve warm.

Nutrition: Calories: 69; Fat: 4 gm; Carbs: 1 gm; Fiber: 0.1 gm; Protein: 6 gm

18. Ginger, Mushroom and Cauliflower Broth

Preparation Time: ten mins

Cooking Time: fifty mins

Servings: three

Ingredients:

- one big yellow onion
- one teacup celery stalks, severed
- two carrots, cubed or cubed
- 10 French beans
- 1 ginger root, skinned, cubed, or grated
- 1-2 stalks celery leaves or coriander leaves
- one and half teacups mushrooms, sliced

- 8 cauliflower florets
- one tsp garlic, severed
- one tbsp oil
- 1 stalk spring green onion
- half tsp crushed pepper or ground pepper

Directions:

1. Transfer the entire components to your stockpot. Top with sufficient water to cover. Then, allow slowly come to a boil on high heat.
2. Switch to low heat. Simmer for almost fifty mins.
3. Set and pour the mixture through a fine-mesh strainer into a big container. Taste and season with salt.
4. Serve warm.
5. Relish!

Nutrition: Calories: 141; Fat: 5 gm; Carbs: 22 gm; Fiber: 7 gm; Protein: 5 gm

19. Fish Broth

Preparation Time: fifteen mins

Cooking Time: forty-five mins

Servings: three

Ingredients:

- one big onion, severed
- one big carrot severed
- one fennel bulb and fronds, severed (optional)
- 3 celery stalks, severed
- Salt
- 2-5 pounds fish bones and heads
- 1 handful dried mushrooms (optional)
- 2-4 bay leaves
- 1-star anise pod (optional)
- one-two tsps thyme, dried or fresh
- three to four pieces dried kombu kelp (optional)

Directions:

1. Transfer the bones and vegetables to your stockpot. Top with sufficient water to cover. Then, allow slowly come to a boil on high heat.
2. Set to low heat. Simmer for forty-five mins.
3. Set and pour the mixture through a fine-mesh strainer into a big container. Taste and season with salt.
4. Serve warm.
5. Relish!

Nutrition: Calories: 29; Fat: 1 gm; Carbs: 2 gm; Fiber: 1 gm; Protein: 1 gm

20. Clear Pumpkin Broth

Preparation Time: fifteen mins

Cooking Time: thirty mins

Servings: six

Ingredients:

- six teacups water

- two tbsps ginger, crushed
- two teacups potatoes, skinned and cubed
- three teacups kabocha, skinned and cubed
- one carrot, skinned and cubed
- one onion, cubed
- half teacup scallions, severed

Directions:

1. Transfer the bones and vegetables to your stockpot. Top with sufficient water to cover. Then, allow slowly come to a boil on high heat.
2. Switch to low heat. Simmer for almost thirty mins.
3. Set and pour the mixture through a fine-mesh strainer into a big container. Taste and season with salt.
4. Serve warm.
5. Relish!

Nutrition: Calories: 216; Fat: 1 gm; Carbs: 37 gm; Fiber: 4 gm; Protein: 8 gm

21. Pork Stock

Preparation Time: fifteen mins

Cooking Time: twelve hrs

Servings: eight

Ingredients:

- two lbs. pork bones, roasted
- 1 onion, severed in quarters
- two celery stalks, severed in half
- 2 carrots, severed in half
- 3 whole garlic pieces
- two bay leaves
- one tbsp salt
- Filtered water (enough to cover bones)

Directions:

1. Transfer the bones and vegetables to your stockpot. Top with sufficient water to cover. Then, allow slowly come to a boil on high heat.
2. Set to low heat and simmer for twelve hrs.
3. Set and pour the mixture through a fine-mesh strainer into a big container. Taste and season with salt.
4. Serve warm.
5. Relish!

Nutrition: Calories: 69; Fat: 4 gm; Carbs: 1 gm; Fiber: 0.1 gm; Protein: 6 gm

22. Slow Cooker Pork Bone Broth

Preparation Time: fifteen mins

Cooking Time: twenty-four hrs

Servings: twelve

Ingredients:

- two lbs. pork bones, roasted
- 1/2 onion, severed
- two medium carrots, severed

- 1 stalk celery, severed
- 2 whole garlic pieces
- 1 bay leaf
- one tbsp sea salt
- one tsp peppercorns
- quarter teacup apple cider vinegar
- Filtered water (enough to cover bones)

Directions:

1. Transfer the entire components to your slow cooker. Top with sufficient water to cover. Then, allow slowly come to a boil on high heat.
2. Switch to low heat. Simmer for almost twenty-four hrs.
3. Set and pour the mixture through a fine-mesh strainer into a big container. Taste and season with salt.
4. Serve warm.
5. Relish!

Nutrition: Calories: 65; Fat: 2 gm; Carbs: 7 gm; Fiber: 4 gm; Protein: 6 gm

23. Strawberry Overnight Oats

Preparation Time: five mins

Cooking Time: zero mins

Total time: five mins

Servings: one

Ingredients:

- half teacup (50 grams) rolled or old-fashioned oats. Use certified gluten-free oats if necessary.
- one tbsp chia
- three-quarter teacup (180 ml) non-dairy milk
- half tsp vanilla extract
- one tbsp maple syrup (optional). Use real maple syrup, not pancake syrup.
- one tbsp strawberry jam (optional - but recommended)
- Around half teacup (60 grams) fresh strawberries, severed

Directions:

1. Include the oats and chia to a jar (or another covered container).
2. Stir in the milk, vanilla extract, and optional maple syrup.
3. Pour in the strawberry jam, followed by the strawberries.
4. Place the container in the fridge for almost 3 to four hrs but up to seventy-two hrs is ok.
5. Eat the oats straight from the jar, or transfer them to a container beforehand.

Nutrition: Calories: 388; Carbohydrates: 61 gm; Protein: 14 gm; Fat: 10 gm; Cholesterol: 386 mg

24. Ginger Peach Smoothie

Preparation Time: five mins

Cooking Time: five mins

Total time: ten mins

Servings: one

Ingredients:

- two ripe, juicy peaches, (you can use frozen peaches, but if you do, use a fresh banana and not a frozen one)
- one medium frozen banana (fresh or frozen)
- three-quarter teacup (180 ml) non-dairy milk
- one tbsp maple syrup, as required
- 1 approximately two and half inches long stick fresh ginger, roughly x half inch wide, or quarter to half tsp ground ginger

Directions:

1. Take out the pits from the peaches. Blend them with the rest of the components in a blender. I recommend using only half of the fresh ginger or 14 teaspoons of ground ginger, to begin.
2. Blend till smooth; then, taste it. If you want a stronger flavor, include a little more ginger.
3. Serve immediately.

Nutrition: Calories: 337; Carbohydrates: 72 gm; Protein: 9 gm; Fat: 4 gm; Cholesterol: 186 mg

25. Strawberry Banana Peanut Butter Smoothie

Preparation Time: five mins

Cooking Time: five mins

Total time: ten mins

Servings: one

Ingredients:

- two teacups (approx. 288 grams) strawberries, fresh or frozen
- one medium frozen banana, fresh and not frozen (if using frozen strawberries)
- two tbsps peanut butter, or any other nut butter
- one teacup (240 ml) plant milk, your choice

Optional:

- one tbsp maple syrup, or a Medjool date
- one tbsp flax
- one tbsp chia

Directions:

1. Inside a mixer, blend the components.
2. Blend till entirely smooth.
3. Check the sweetness, and if required, include the optional maple syrup or date. Then, mix again to blend.

Nutrition: Calories: 465; Carbohydrates: 60 gm; Protein: 18 gm; Fat: 21 gm; Cholesterol: 276 mg

26. Granola

Preparation Time: five mins

Cooking Time: twenty mins

Total time: twenty-five mins

Servings: six

Ingredients:

- two teacups (180 grams) rolled or old-fashioned oats. Use certified gluten-free for gluten-free granola)
- one teacup (85 grams) raw almonds your choice, pecans, walnuts, etc. (or more pumpkin or sunflower for nut-free)
- half teacup (80 grams) shelled pumpkin, sunflower or hemp, or a mix of all 3
- half teacup (25 grams) puffed rice, optional. It adds fantastic texture - if you don't use it, make up the quantity with more oats
- 6 tablespoons creamy butter, your choice
- three-quarter teacup (180 ml) brown rice syrup or maple syrup. Brown rice syrup will give you bigger clusters
- half tsp fine sea salt (if you use iodized-table salt instead, you will need to use less)
- one tsp ground cinnamon
- one tsp vanilla extract
- one teacup dried raisins, sultanas, cranberries, tart cherries or chocolate chips, or any other dried fruit (severed if it's something like apricots or dates)

Directions:

1. Warm up the oven to 350 deg.F (175 deg.C), and place a shelf on the bottom level.
2. Using parchment paper, or a silicone baking mat. Line a big baking pot.
3. Include the oats and optional puffed rice to a big blending container. To mix, stir all collectively.
4. Inside a medium blending container, blend the butter, syrup, salt, cinnamon, and vanilla extract. To mix, whisk everything together.
5. Pour the wet mixture into the oat mixture, and stir with a wooden spoon or spatula till everything is mixed, moist, and sticky.
6. Spread it evenly over the prepared tray, about 3/4 inch deep.
7. Bake for ten mins on the lowest oven shelf. Then, take from the oven and stir with a spatula, to ensure equal cooking. After you've finished swirling it, firmly press it all over with a spatula or the bottom of a cup. This helps it cling and forms wonderful big clumps when crumbled later.
8. Return to the oven and bake for an extra ten-fifteen mins, or till the top is brown and the house smells toasty.
9. Take out from the oven. Spray the dried fruit/chocolate chips; then, leave to cool fully on the baking tray. As it cools, the granola will solidify.
10. Break up the granola into chunky pieces with your hands. Place it in a sealed container. It will last 6 to 8 weeks.

Nutrition: Calories: 250; Carbohydrates: 35 gm; Protein: 8 gm; Fat: 13 gm; Cholesterol: 621 mg

27. Persimmon Smoothie

Preparation Time: five mins

Cooking Time: five mins

Total time: ten mins

Servings: one

Ingredients:

- two medium ripe persimmons
- one medium frozen banana
- one teacup dairy-free milk
- About 10 cashews (if you don't have a high-powered blender, soak the cashew in hot water for five mins prior to adding it to the blender). See notes for cashew alternatives.
- quarter tsp cinnamon (include a little more if you prefer a stronger cinnamon taste)
- one tbsp maple syrup

Directions:

1. Take out and discard the persimmon leaves. Then, chop each fruit into pieces. Blend them with the rest of the components, except for the maple syrup, till smooth.
2. Use the blender to give it a brief taste and, if required, include the maple syrup. After adding it, give it a brisk 5-second mix prior to serving.

Nutrition: Calories: 298; Carbohydrates: 41 gm; Protein: 11 gm; Fat: 12 gm; Cholesterol: 121 mg

28. Cranberry Smoothie

Preparation Time: five mins

Cooking Time: zero mins

Total time: five mins

Servings: one

Ingredients:

- 75 gm / three-quarter teacup frozen cranberries (or fresh cranberries but include a handful of ice too)
- one big apple, cored and severed into chunks
- 1 small handful / about two tbsps raw pecans or walnuts (see notes for nut-free option)
- one tbsp maple syrup
- 240 ml / one teacup non-dairy milk
- quarter tsp ground cinnamon

Directions:

1. Include the components to a blender.
2. Blend till smooth.

Nutrition: Calories: 424; Carbohydrates: 61 gm; Protein: 10 gm; Fat: 19 gm; Cholesterol: 251 mg

29. Kale Apple Smoothie

Preparation Time: five mins

Cooking Time: five mins

Total time: ten mins

Servings: one

Ingredients:

- two big kale leaves, washed with stems taken out. Use a couple of handfuls of baby kale instead for a milder kale flavor
- one big apple, cored (no need to peel unless you want to).
- one tbsp chia
- two tsps ground flax or whole flax
- one - two tbsps maple syrup
- half medium lemon, juice only
- 180mls / three-quarter teacup plant-based milk, include up to a quarter teacup more to thin the smoothie if you prefer it that way
- five ice cubes, optional but will make it colder and a bit thicker
- one tbsp almond butter, optional – it's great with or without

Directions:

1. Blend the entire components in a blender till smooth. On my Blendtec, I use the smoothie option.
2. Check the sweetness and, if required, include a bit more maple syrup.
3. Serve instantly.

Nutrition: Calories: 319; Carbohydrates: 63 gm; Protein: 9 gm; Fat: 7 gm; Cholesterol: 266 mg

30. Glowing Skin Smoothie

Preparation Time: five mins

Cooking Time: five mins

Total time: ten mins

Servings: two

Ingredients:

- quarter teacup cashew pieces or 1 very heaping quarter teacup of whole ones about 38 gm
- one teacup 240 ml water or coconut water for an extra skin boost!
- one medium banana
- 1 very heaping cup frozen mango pieces around 140 gm, see recipe notes if you only have fresh mango
- one tbsp chia, optional
- one-eighth tsp vanilla bean powder or half tsp vanilla extract
- half tsp ground cardamom
- quarter tsp ground turmeric

- one-eighth tsp ground ginger or a small piece of fresh ginger
- one tbsp maple syrup or one big Medjool date

Directions:

1. If you don't have a high-powered blender, soak the cashew in boiling water for fifteen mins or cold water for two hrs (this technique will maintain the nutrients); then, drain.
2. Blend the cashew with the water in a blender till smooth. You've just created cashew milk!
3. Include the other components, and mix till smooth.
4. Serve with a decorative sprinkling of cardamom and turmeric, if desired.

Nutrition: Calories: 342; Carbohydrates: 70 gm; Protein: 8 gm; Fat: 15 gm; Cholesterol: 82 mg

31. Cranberry Sauce

Preparation Time: five mins

Cooking Time: fifteen mins

Total time: twenty mins

Servings: sixteen

Ingredients:

- 24 oz. / 680 gm fresh or frozen cranberries
- half teacup / 100 gm sugar, granulated white or cane sugar
- half teacup / 120 ml maple syrup (real, natural maple syrup, not pancake syrup)
- ⅓ cup / 80 ml vegan red wine or port, or orange juice for an alcohol-free alternative
- one big orange, zest, and juice
- one medium cinnamon stick
- 1 approximately 3-inch piece of fresh rosemary

Directions:

To make on the stovetop:

1. Wash the cranberries, and take out the soft ones. One teacup of them should be put away, and the rest should be blended with everything else in a medium saucepan. Cook, frequently stirring, at middling temp. till the sauce thickens and becomes jammy. The cranberries should break down. Usually, it takes approximately fifteen mins.
2. Take out the rosemary and cinnamon stick from the pan. Set aside. Take a quick taste, but be careful because it will be extremely hot. If you want to include more sugar, do so now because it will dissolve in the heat. But, keep in mind that it's intended as required tart.
3. Stir in the cranberries that have been put away. The residual heat will cook them sufficiently prior to the sauce cools, giving them a good texture.
4. Allow cooling entirely prior to transferring to sterilized jars or freezer-safe containers.

To make in an instant pot:

1. Wash the cranberries and take out the soft ones. Scoop out approximately one teacup and put away till the end. Place the rest of the components in the instant pot.

2. Stir in the sugar, maple syrup, red wine, orange juice, and zest. On top, place the cinnamon stick and rosemary.

3. Close the vent and replace the cover on the instant pot. Cook for three mins on high pressure prior to allowing the pressure to naturally release. Open the lid, once the pin has dropped. Don't be alarmed if it appears frothy and unappealing. Take out the cinnamon stick and rosemary. Then, stir in the saved cranberries. The rest of the heat is sufficient to cook them. Stir everything thoroughly. It now looks better. Take a short sip. Be cautious since it will be quite hot. If you find it too sour, include a bit of extra sugar now since it will dissolve in the heat. But, keep in mind that a little bit of acidity is excellent since it pairs well with your meals.

4. Allow cooling entirely prior to using. At this stage, the lid can be on or off, although it will cool faster with the cover off. Decant into jars or freezer-safe containers, once cold.

Nutrition: Calories: 74; Carbohydrates: 18 gm; Protein: 1 gm; Fat: 1 gm; Cholesterol: 80 mg

32. Chocolate Tahini Pumpkin Smoothie

Preparation Time: five mins

Cooking Time: zero mins

Total time: five mins

Servings: one

Ingredients:

- one frozen banana
- one tbsp cocoa
- eight tbsps / half teacup pumpkin puree, canned or fresh
- one mildly heaping tbsp Tahini
- two tbsps maple syrup
- 180 ml / three-quarter teacup non-dairy milk

Directions:

1. Include the entire components to a blender.
2. Blend till entirely smooth.
3. Serve immediately.

Nutrition: Calories: 383; Carbohydrates: 73 gm; Protein: 7 gm; Fat: 11 gm; Cholesterol: 32 mg

33. Caramel Sauce

Preparation Time: two mins

Cooking Time: three mins

Total time: five mins

Servings: four

Ingredients:

- 100 gm / half teacup coconut sugar

- two tbsps water
- two tbsps Tahini (see recipe note)
- two tbsps vegan butter or coconut oil (solid measurement)
- one-eighth to quarter tsp salt

Directions:

1. Inside a saucepot, blend the coconut sugar and water.
2. Cook at middling temp. till the sugar has fully melted, and the mixture is just beginning to bubble. Don't stir!! Swirl the pan a little, if necessary. It will take no more than two to three mins. If you leave it unattended for too long, it will quickly burn.
3. Take the pan off the heat and stir in the Tahini, salt, and vegan butter or coconut oil. Stir vigorously till everything is fully incorporated. It's natural to see a few bright specks through it. If you're having problems getting it to come together, place it back at low temp. for thirty secs.

Nutrition: Calories: 195; Carbohydrates: 25 gm; Protein: 1 gm; Fat: 10 gm; Cholesterol: 156 mg

34. Lemon Cheesecake Smoothie

Preparation Time: five mins

Cooking Time: five mins

Total time: ten mins

Servings: two

Ingredients:

- one medium juicy lemon
- one teacup (240 ml) light canned coconut milk
- ¼ heaping cup (50 grams) cooked chickpeas
- 1 to 2 Medjool dates
- quarter teacup (25 grams) severed pecan measured in pieces, not whole
- one teacup (150 grams) frozen mango pieces
- quarter tsp ground turmeric
- quarter tsp salt
- half tsp apple cider vinegar
- one tbsp maple syrup optional

Directions:

1. To begin, zest the lemon. Blend the lemon zest; then, take out the rest of the peel and pith (the white stuff) from the lemon. I do this by cutting both sharp ends of the lemon, and then standing it up on the board. Then, with a sharp knife, slice around it, just deep enough to take out the pit while leaving the flesh intact.

2. After that, place the entire lemon in the blender and take out the pit, and peel.

3. Except for the maple syrup, blend the entire of the components inside a blending container.

4. Blend till the mixture is smooth. It yields a dense smoothie. If you like it a little thinner, include a little extra coconut milk or a drop of water to thin it out.

5. If you want a little extra sweetness, include a little more maple syrup. It goes well with maple syrup. Blend for a second on low to disperse, then pour into a glass and serve.

Nutrition: Calories: 549; Carbohydrates: 68 gm; Protein: 6 gm; Fat: 39 gm; Cholesterol: 140 mg

35. <u>**Double Chocolate Scones**</u>

Preparation Time: ten mins

Cooking Time: twenty-five mins

Total time: thirty-five mins

Servings: eight

Ingredients:

- 125 gm / one teacup all-purpose flour
- 97 gm / three-quarter teacup whole-wheat flour
- 25 gm / quarter teacup cocoa powder
- 62 gm / quarter heaping cup natural cane sugar
- half tsp salt
- one tbsp ground flax
- one tbsp baking powder
- quarter cup coconut oil (it needs to be hard)
- one tsp vanilla extract
- 207 ml / three-quarter teacup + two tbsps cup of non-dairy milk
- 130 g / three-quarter teacup dairy-free chocolate chips or chunks
- A little sugar for sprinkling

For the drizzle (optional)

- 43 gm quarter teacup dairy-free chocolate
- two tbsps non-dairy milk

Directions:

1. Warm up the oven to 400 deg.F.
2. Use parchment paper or a silicone baking mat to line a baking sheet.
3. Inside a big mixing basin, blend the flour and baking powder.
4. Mix in the coconut oil with your fingertips or a pastry cutter till the mixture resembles bread crumbs.
5. Stir in the entire rest of the dry components, including the chocolate.
6. Include the vanilla extract to the milk and mix to blend, then include the liquid to the dry components and swirl to blend.
7. It's now simpler to get your hands into the dough and shape it into a ball.
8. Place on the prepared tray and press or roll into a 1 inch dense round.

9. Divide the mixture into eight similar wedges and divide them so that they all have some space between them.
10. Spray with sugar and bake for twenty to twenty-five mins, or till thoroughly cooked.
11. Allow cooling on a cooling rack.
12. For the optional chocolate drizzling, put the chocolate and milk in a small dish and gently melt in a microwave or over a saucepan of boiling water.
13. Spray the melted chocolate mixture over the cooled scones using a spoon.

Nutrition: Calories: 285; Carbohydrates: 41 gm; Protein: 6 gm; Fat: 12 gm; Cholesterol: 90 mg

36. <u>**Chocolate Ice Cream**</u>

Preparation Time: five mins

Cooking Time: one min

Total time: six mins

Servings: four

Ingredients:

- four bananas ripened and frozen
- quarter teacup organic cocoa powder
- one tbsp organic vanilla extract
- one tbsp coconut milk or another dairy-free milk (optional)

Directions:

1. Frozen bananas should be cut into pieces. Put everything inside a blending container or blender. Blend till the mixture is crumbly.
2. Mix in the chocolate powder and vanilla extract. Blend till everything is properly blended. In the food processor, it will form a ball.
3. If the mixture needs additional liquid to blend effectively, include coconut milk or another dairy-free milk.

Nutrition: Calories: 128; Carbohydrates: 30 gm; Protein: 2 gm; Fat: 1 gm; Cholesterol: 13 mg

37. <u>**Healthy Watermelon Popsicles**</u>

Preparation Time: ten mins

Cooking Time: one hundred and eighty mins

Total time: one hundred and ninety mins

Servings: four

Ingredients:

- two teacups watermelon cubed
- one teacup strawberries hulled and halved
- two tbsps vegan chocolate chips or raisins
- quarter teacup coconut milk (full fat) plus two tbsps
- 2 kiwis, skinned and cubed

Directions:

1. Watermelon should be cut and cubed. Strawberries should be de-stemmed and sliced into quarters. Blend the two teacups of watermelon and one teacup of

strawberries in a big blending container till smooth. Fill four popsicle molds about 3/4 full with the mixture.

2. Divide the chocolate chips equally between the four molds. Gently press the chocolate chips into the molds with a popsicle stick, spreading them evenly. Raisins can also be used.

3. Freeze for one hour or till frozen.

4. While the first is frozen, blend 1four teacups coconut milk and one tsp maple syrup. After the initial layer has hardened, equally distribute the coconut milk among the four molds, about one tbsp each mold.

5. Freeze for one further hour or till set.

6. While the second layer is freezing, take out the kiwi's outer covering and slice it into tiny bits. Blend with two tbsps coconut milk.

7. Pour the kiwi layer on top of the coconut layer after it has set. Freeze for an extra hour or till set. Serve and have fun!

Nutrition: Calories: 174; Carbohydrates: 26 gm; Protein: 3 gm; Fat: 9 gm; Cholesterol: 356 mg

38. **Spinach Mango Vegan Popsicles**

Preparation Time: five mins

Cooking Time: one hundred and eighty mins

Total time: one hundred and eighty-five mins

Servings: four

Ingredients:

- one teacup unsweetened almond milk
- one and half teacups fresh spinach
- ⅓ cup unsweetened coconut milk yogurt
- half teacup frozen mango
- half teacup frozen banana optional
- two tbsps maple syrup optional

Directions:

1. Blend almond milk and spinach in a blender. Blend on medium-high till the spinach is thoroughly broken down and incorporated.

2. Blend the coconut milk, mango, banana (optional), and maple syrup inside a blending container. Blend till entirely smooth.

3. Fill popsicle molds with the mixture. Popsicle sticks should be inserted. If they don't stand straight in the molds, place them in the freezer for an hour prior to inserting them.

4. For best results, freeze for almost three hrs, preferably overnight.

Nutrition: Calories: 81; Carbohydrates: 15 gm; Protein: 1 gm; Fat: 1 gm; Cholesterol: 253 mg

39. **Mango Banana Smoothie**

Preparation Time: five mins

Cooking Time: zero mins

Total time: five mins

Servings: two

Ingredients:

- one teacup frozen cubed mango
- one frozen banana severed
- one teacup unsweetened almond milk
- quarter teacup dairy-free coconut milk yogurt plain unsweetened
- 1 scoop pea protein powder optional

Directions:

1. Fill your blender or smoothie cup with almond milk, coconut yogurt, protein powder, fresh mangoes, and severed frozen banana in the following order: almond milk, coconut yogurt, protein powder, fresh mangoes, and severed frozen banana.

2. Connect the blender lid or the smoothie attachment blade. Begin on low and gradually increase speed till all items are thoroughly mixed.

3. Pour the mixture into two glasses. Serve with fresh mango, chia, and coconut flakes on top (optional)

Nutrition: Calories: 193; Carbohydrates: 30 gm; Protein: 14 gm; Fat: 1 gm; Cholesterol: 318 mg

40. **Spinach Blueberry Smoothie**

Preparation Time: three mins

Cooking Time: two mins

Total time: five mins

Servings: one

Ingredients:

- one teacup almond milk unsweetened vanilla or regular
- one teacup raw spinach loosely packed
- one frozen banana severed into chunks
- half teacup frozen blueberries
- one tbsp chia

Directions:

1. Inside a mixer, blend the components in the sequence listed in the recipe, beginning with the almond milk and working your way up to the spinach, frozen banana, frozen blueberries, and chia.

2. Blend till entirely smooth.

Nutrition: Calories: 247; Carbohydrates: 45 gm; Protein: 6 gm; Fat: 1 gm; Cholesterol: 261 mg

41. **Snowman Christmas Smoothie**

Preparation Time: five mins

Cooking Time: zero mins

Total time: five mins

Servings: two

Ingredients:

- 1 banana frozen and severed
- one teacup unsweetened almond milk

- quarter teacup desiccated coconut shredded, unsweetened
- half teacup coconut whipped cream optional
- Blue sugar sprinkles optional

Directions:
1. Assemble the snowman cups. To construct the mouth, draw two circular eyes, one triangular nose, and 5-6 tiny circles in a curved shape.
2. Inside a mixer, blend the almond milk, banana, and coconut.
3. Blend till entirely smooth. Approximately 5-10 seconds
4. Pour the smoothie into the glasses. Spray with blue sugar sprinkles and top with coconut whipped cream.

Nutrition: Calories: 51; Carbohydrates: 17 gm; Protein: 8 gm; Fat: 6 gm; Cholesterol: 201 mg

42. **Clean Green Shamrock Shake**

Preparation Time: five mins

Cooking Time: zero mins

Total time: five mins

Servings: one

Ingredients:
- one teacup light coconut milk
- ¼ avocado
- 1 banana frozen
- half teacup fresh leaf spinach
- ⅛ tablespoon peppermint extract
- one tbsp dairy-free chocolate chips optional

Directions:
1. Inside a mixer, blend the frozen banana, coconut milk, avocado, spinach, and peppermint essence. Blend till smooth and well blended.
2. Fill a glass halfway with ice and top with chocolate chunks.

Nutrition: Calories: 382; Carbohydrates: 41 gm; Protein: 3 gm; Fat: 23 gm; Cholesterol: 183 mg

43. **Pumpkin Smoothie**

Preparation Time: three mins

Cooking Time: zero mins

Total time: three mins

Servings: two

Ingredients:
- one banana frozen
- half teacup pumpkin puree
- one teacup almond milk unsweetened
- half tsp pumpkin pie spice
- one tbsp maple syrup optional
- half teacup ice cubes

Directions:

1. Inside a mixer, blend the frozen banana, pumpkin purée, almond milk, pumpkin pie spice, and maple syrup.
2. Blend till the mixture is smooth and creamy. If using a high-speed blender, start at the lowest level and gradually increase to 5 or 6 till all components are incorporated. Blend in the ice till well mixed.
3. Pour the mixture into two glasses. Serve with a sprinkling of pumpkin pie spice on top.

Nutrition: Calories: 119; Carbohydrates: 26 gm; Protein: 2 gm; Fat: 1 gm; Cholesterol: 19 mg

Lunch

44. **Banana Oat Shake**

Preparation Time: twenty mins

Cooking Time: zero mins

Total time: twenty mins

Servings: two

Ingredients:
- half teacup cooked oatmeal, chilled
- two-third teacup skim milk
- two tbsps brown sugar
- one tbsp wheat germ
- one and half tsps vanilla extract
- 1/2 frozen banana, cut into chunks

Directions:
1. Blend the oatmeal for a couple of mins in a blender.
2. Mix in the milk, brown sugar, wheat germ, vanilla extract, and 1/2 banana. Blend till the mixture is dense and smooth.
3. If desired, serve with ice.

Nutrition: Calories: 173; Carbohydrates: 33 gm; Protein: 6 gm; Fat: 1 gm; Cholesterol: 150 mg

45. **Banana-Apple Smoothie**

Preparation Time: fifteen mins

Cooking Time: zero mins

Total time: fifteen mins

Servings: one

Ingredients:
- 1/2 banana, skinned and cut into chunks
- half teacup plain yogurt
- half teacup unsweetened applesauce
- quarter teacup skim milk
- one tbsp honey
- two tbsps oat bran

Directions:
1. Inside a mixer, blend the banana, yogurt, applesauce, milk, and honey.
2. Blend till entirely smooth.
3. Blend in the oat bran till it is thickened.

Nutrition: Calories: 292; Carbohydrates: 61 gm; Protein: 9 gm; Fat: 17 gm; Cholesterol: 103 mg

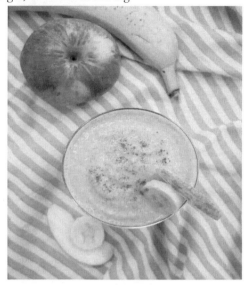

46. Berrylicious Smoothie

Preparation Time: twenty mins

Cooking Time: zero mins

Total time: twenty mins

Servings: two

Ingredients:

- quarter teacup cranberry juice cocktail
- two-third teacup silken tofu, firm
- half teacup raspberries, frozen, unsweetened
- half teacup blueberries, frozen, unsweetened
- one tsp vanilla extract
- half tsp powdered lemonade, such as country time

Directions:

1. Fill a blender halfway with juice.
2. Blend the rest of the components.
3. Blend till entirely smooth.
4. Serve immediately and relish!

Nutrition: Calories: 115; Carbohydrates: 18 gm; Protein: 6 gm; Fat: 3 gm; Cholesterol: 223 mg

47. Buttermilk Herb Ranch Dressing

Preparation Time: ten mins

Cooking Time: zero mins

Total time: ten mins

Servings: two

Ingredients:

- half teacup mayonnaise
- half teacup milk
- two tbsps vinegar
- one tbsp fresh chives, severed
- one tbsp dill
- one tbsp oregano leaves, severed
- quarter tsp garlic powder

Directions:

1. In a medium mixing dish, blend mayonnaise, milk, and vinegar.
2. Then, with quarter tsp garlic powder, include fresh chives, dill, and oregano leaves.
3. Blend everything.
4. Allow almost one hour for flavors to emerge.
5. Before serving, thoroughly mix the dressing.

Nutrition: Calories: 83; Carbohydrates: 1 gm; Protein: 1 gm; Fat: 6 gm; Cholesterol: 64 mg

48. Citrus Relish

Preparation Time: ten mins

Cooking Time: two mins

Total time: twelve mins

Servings: eight

Ingredients:

- two lbs. small lemons, limes, kumquats, or oranges
- one quart white vinegar
- quarter teacup mustard
- Glass jars
- 2-4 tablespoons sugar

Directions:

Pickled fruit:

1. At the stem end of each fruit, make a cross. Quarter the oranges if using.
2. Fill glass jars halfway with vinegar.
3. To each jar, include two tbsps of mustard. Put on the lids.
4. Allow it to sit at room temp. for around a month prior to preparing the relish listed below and serving.

Citrus relish:

1. In a small frying pan, blend the fruit and sugar: include additional sugar as required.
2. For five-ten mins, shake the pan often at middling temp. till the mixture boils and the fruit turns glossy and transparent.
3. Serve hot or cold.
4. The vinegar leftover from the pickled fruit can be used to make salad dressing or to marinate chicken or seafood.

Nutrition: Calories: 26; Carbohydrates: 7 gm; Protein: 0 gm; Fat: 0 gm; Cholesterol: 37 mg

49. Chickpea Pancakes Recipe

Preparation Time: ten mins

Cooking Time: fifteen mins

Total time: twenty-five mins

Servings: twenty-three

Ingredients:

- one teacup (120 gm) chickpea flour
- one and half teacups (375 ml) water
- two tbsps olive oil *see note 1
- 1 carrot, finely grated
- 1/4 red capsicum, finely severed
- one spring onion, finely severed
- quarter tbsp turmeric
- quarter tbsp cumin
- two tbsps severed coriander (cilantro)
- quarter tbsp salt

Directions:

1. Inside a blending basin, blend the chickpea flour and water, constantly stirring to create a smooth, lump-free batter. Set aside.
2. Warm half tbsp of the oil in a frying pan at medium-high temp. Blend the carrot, onion, turmeric, and cumin inside a blending container. Reduce the heat to medium-low and continue to simmer till the vegetables are softened (around four-five mins).
3. Blend the carrot mixture, severed coriander, and salt in the chickpea batter (if using). Stir till everything is well mixed.
4. At medium-high temp., heat a nonstick frying pan. When the pan is heated, pour in the olive oil (or use spray oil). Place a tablespoon of butter in the pan and spread it out with the back of your spoon (to make them thinner). To fill the pan, repeat the process.
5. Cook each side for around two mins (this will vary depending on the pan, heat, and how thin your pancake is). Look for bubbles to develop (as seen above), and your pancakes should be able to be easily flipped.
6. Take out the pancakes from the pan and continue with the rest of the batter.

Nutrition: Calories: 32; Carbohydrates: 3 gm; Protein: 1 gm; Fat: 1 gm; Cholesterol: 27 mg

50. Red Wine Sangria Recipe

Preparation Time: fifteen mins

Cooking Time: fifteen mins

Total time: thirty mins

Servings: eight

Ingredients:

- 750 ml Rioja wine
- three-quarter teacup Solerno blood orange liqueur
- three-quarter teacup Leblon Cachaca Brazilian rum
- one and half teacups orange juice
- three-quarter teacup cherry juice
- three-quarter teacup simple syrup sugar syrup
- half teacup fresh lime juice
- one and half teacups watermelon balls

- one teacup raspberries
- one teacup blackberries
- 2 mandarin oranges, sliced
- 1 lime, sliced
- 1 bunch basil leaves

Directions:

1. Stir together the entire liquid components in a big pitcher. Then, to the pitcher, include the fresh fruit.
2. Refrigerate for almost two hrs, covered. Pour into glasses and garnish with fresh basil leaves when ready to serve.

Nutrition: Calories: 360; Carbohydrates: 51 gm; Protein: 1 gm; Fat: 1 gm; Cholesterol: 423 mg

51. Salty Dog Cocktail Recipe

Preparation Time: three mins

Cooking Time: zero mins

Total time: three mins

Servings: two

Ingredients:

- 4 oz. ruby red grapefruit juice
- 2 oz. vodka
- 1 oz. club soda or sparkling grapefruit-flavored water
- one-two tsps simple syrup
- Ice

For garnish:

- Kosher salt or Fleur de Sel agave syrup, grapefruit wedges

Directions:

1. Set out two tiny shallow plates for the salt rim. In one plate, spread salt, and in the other, spread a thin layer of agave syrup (or just syrup). Dip the edge of a highball glass in the syrup prior to dipping it in the salt.
2. Fill the glass three-quarters full of ice for each cocktail. Blend the grapefruit juice, vodka, club soda, and one tsp simple syrup inside a blending container.
3. Use a cocktail swizzle stick to stir. If desired, include a bit extra simple syrup as required. Serve with a fresh grapefruit slice on the rim.

Note: Include a sprinkle of cayenne to the salt prior to dipping for a fiery salty dog.

Nutrition: Calories: 202; Carbohydrates: 18 gm; Protein: 1 gm; Fat: 11 gm; Cholesterol: 26 mg

52. Simple Syrup

Preparation Time: two mins

Cooking Time: three mins

Total time: five mins

Servings: eight

Ingredients:

- one teacup water

- one teacup granulated sugar or turbinado, demerara

Directions:

1. Heat a small saucepot on high. Fill the saucepan halfway with water and sugar.
2. Raise to a boil, stirring constantly. Once boiling, take out from heat and stir. (If using herbs for infusion, include them to the simple boiling syrup.)
3. Allow cooling to room temp. prior to storing in a sealed container.

Nutrition: Calories: 97; Carbohydrates: 25 gm; Protein: 2 gm; Fat: 12 gm; Cholesterol: 44 mg

53. Rose Sangria Recipe

Preparation Time: fifteen mins

Cooking Time: zero mins

Total time: fifteen mins

Servings: eight

Ingredients:

- 750 ml French rosé wine (1 bottle)
- one teacup pink grapefruit juice
- three-quarter teacup Bourbon
- half teacup honey
- quarter teacup Chambord (raspberry liqueur)
- two teacups watermelon balls
- one and half teacups fresh sliced strawberries
- 6 oz. fresh raspberries

Directions:

1. Scoop two teacups of watermelon balls from a big piece of fresh watermelon using a melon baller. Strawberries, sliced.
2. Inside a big pitcher, blend the rosé wine, grapefruit juice, whiskey, honey, and Chambord. Stir the honey into the mixture till it melts (If your honey is particularly dense, reheat it first to thin it up prior to adding to the recipe.) After that, toss in the watermelon balls and strawberries. Refrigerate for almost two hrs, covered.
3. Stir and taste for sweetness after almost two hours. If you want your sangria sweeter, include a bit, extra honey. If the sangria is too powerful, serve it over ice. When ready to serve, mix in the fresh raspberries and divide among glasses.

Nutrition: Calories: 209; Carbohydrates: 26 gm; Protein: 0 gm; Fat: 0 gm; Cholesterol: 180 mg

54. Champagne Holiday Punch Recipe

Preparation Time: two mins

Cooking Time: five mins

Total time: seven mins

Servings: sixteen

Ingredients:

- 750 ml Champagne (1 bottle)
- 24 oz. ginger beer (2 bottles)

- three teacups cranberry juice cocktail (or juice blend)
- two teacups ruby red grapefruit juice
- one teacup spiced rum, optional
- Possible garnishes: fresh cranberries, grapefruit slices, cinnamon sticks

Directions:

1. All components should be chilled. When ready to serve, blend the entire components in a punch container.
2. Serve with cranberries, grapefruit slices, and cinnamon sticks as garnish.

Nutrition: Calories: 107; Carbohydrates: 13 gm; Protein: 0 gm; Fat: 0 gm; Cholesterol: 0 mg

55. White Sangria

Preparation Time: ten mins

Cooking Time: ten mins

Total time: twenty mins

Servings: ten

Ingredients:

- 750 ml Moscato wine riesling is my second choice
- one and half teacups orange-pineapple juice
- one teacup Domaine de Canton ginger liqueur
- half teacup Midori melon liqueur
- one teacup Cantaloupe balls
- one teacup sliced strawberries
- 2 mandarin oranges sliced
- 1 lime sliced
- 1 liter Club Soda chilled

Directions:

1. Inside a big pitcher, blend the wine, juice, and liqueurs. Refrigerate for almost one hr after adding the fruit.
2. Pour into glasses 2/3 full (scoop in some fruit) and top with club soda when ready to serve. Serve chilled.

Nutrition: Calories: 218; Carbohydrates: 27 gm; Protein: 1 gm; Fat: 1 gm; Cholesterol: 18 mg

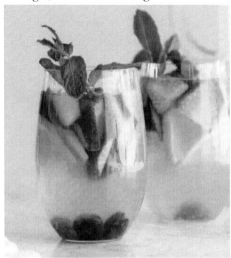

56. Raspberry Mojitos with Basil

Preparation Time: ten mins

Cooking Time: ten mins

Total time: twenty mins

Servings: eight

Ingredients:

- one teacup simple syrup three-quarter teacup sugar + three-quarter teacup water, heated to dissolve
- half teacup torn basil leaves
- one teacup fresh key lime juice. Use regular limes for slightly less acidity.
- one teacup white rum
- quarter teacup Chambord raspberry liquor
- one liter Club Soda
- Ice
- Fresh raspberries and lime slices to garnish

Directions:

1. Inside a big pitcher, blend the simple cooled syrup and the torn basil leaves. Muddle the basil leaves with a big spoon/ladle to unleash their flavor. Beat them up quite hard.
2. Blend the lime juice, rum, and Chambord in a mixing glass. Stir in the club soda and top with ice if the pitcher permits.
3. Garnish each glass with fresh berries and lime slices to serve. Serve cold with or without ice.

Nutrition: Calories: 283; Carbohydrates: 36 gm; Protein: 1 gm; Fat: 1 gm; Cholesterol: 53 mg

57. Margarita Recipe

Preparation Time: ten mins

Cooking Time: ten mins

Total time: twenty mins

Servings: ten

Ingredients:

- 18 oz. tequila Blanco
- 18 oz. fresh-squeezed lime juice. It could be fresh bottled lime juice from the refrigerated section, but not the concentrated kind.
- 9 oz. La Belle or Grand Marnier
- 8 oz. simple syrup + a little extra for glass rims
- 3 oz. orange juice
- 3 oz. triple sec
- Coarse or flaked sea salt for glass rims
- Sliced lime and orange for garnish

Directions:

1. If you don't have any on hand, start by preparing some simple syrup with 7 oz. sugar and 7 oz. water in the microwave till the sugar is entirely melted. You should have around 9-10 oz. leftover for rimming the glasses.
2. Blend the Margarita components in a big pitcher. Chill after thoroughly stirring.
3. Pour the simple leftover syrup into a shallow dish when ready to serve. In a second shallow dish, include sea salt (or flake salt). Then, dip the rims of the glasses in simple syrup, followed by salt.
4. If preferred, include ice to the glasses, and fill a shaker halfway with ice. Shake the margarita mix for 10-15 seconds in a shaker. Pour into serving glasses. Serve the cups garnished with cut limes or oranges. Olé!

Nutrition: Calories: 300; Carbohydrates: 32 gm; Protein: 0 gm; Fat: 0 gm; Cholesterol: 29 mg

58. Grapefruit Basil Sorbet

Preparation Time: thirty-five mins

Cooking Time: twenty mins

Total time: fifty-five mins

Servings: six

Ingredients:

- four big ruby red grapefruits, juiced
- two teacups of water
- one and three-quarter teacups organic cane sugar or palm sugar
- two lemons, zested and juiced
- one teacup basil leaves, packed
- A tweak of salt

Directions:

1. Inside a small saucepot, bring the water and sugar to a boil. When the water is boiling, include the lemon zest, basil leaves, and salt. Take out from the heat and cover with a lid. For almost twenty mins, steep the basil leaves in the simple syrup.
2. Meanwhile, fill a 4-cup measuring pitcher halfway with lemon juice. Juice the grapefruits into the pitcher till 3 glasses of blended juices are measured.

3. Take out the basil leaves and strain the simple syrup. Then blend the syrup and the juice. Refrigerate for almost 2-three hrs (or to speed up, put in the freezer for one hr.)

4. Fill an electric ice cream maker halfway with the sorbet mixture. Turn on and mix for almost twenty mins, or till the mixture achieves a "soft-serve" consistency.

5. Sorbet may be eaten immediately or frozen in a sealed container. Allow the sorbet to soften for ten-fifteen mins after it has been frozen prior to serving.

Note: To achieve the brightest, freshest flavor, use freshly squeezed grapefruits rather than pre-squeezed grapefruit juice.

Nutrition: Calories: 272; Carbohydrates: 70 gm; Protein: 1 gm; Fat: 1 gm; Cholesterol: 38 mg

59. **Bruleed Grapefruit (Pamplemousse Brûlé)**

Preparation Time: five mins

Cooking Time: eight mins

Total time: thirteen mins

Servings: eight

Ingredients:

- four big ripe ruby red grapefruits
- 8 teaspoons granulated sugar
- Brulee Torch

Directions:

1. Place your index finger on the top of a grapefruit stem, and cup your palm around it, from top to bottom. Then, cut it in half in the middle. If you don't notice a floral pattern, you've severed the grapefruit incorrectly. Cut each grapefruit in this manner.

2. I am using a tiny serrated knife cut along the inside rim of each grapefruit half, to separate the fruit from the skin. Then, cut along the membrane between each small triangle section so that each mouthful comes out easily with a spoon. Keep everything intact.

3. Spray one tsp of granulated sugar over the top of each grapefruit half, one at a time. Then, hold the flame over the grapefruit; and, brulee the top till the sugar turns golden and has candied the top of each half. This should take 30-60 seconds per half. Serve immediately and repeat.

Nutrition: Calories: 67; Carbohydrates: 12 gm; Protein: 2 gm; Fat: 2 gm; Cholesterol: 86 mg

60. **Frozen Beers Recipe**

Preparation Time: five mins

Cooking Time: five mins

Total time: ten mins

Servings: two

Ingredients:

- 3 oz. Tequila Blanco
- 1 oz. Triple Sec (orange liqueur)
- 3 oz. fresh lime juice
- 3 oz. simple syrup
- 2 oz. orange juice
- 14 oz. Corona Mexican beer, such as two 7-ounce bottles or one 12-ounce can, any Mexican beer
- three-four teacups ice

Directions:

Self-serve method

1. Inside a mixer, blend tequila, triple sec, lime juice, simple syrup, and orange juice. Pour with 3 glasses of ice. Puree the mixture till it is smooth and foamy. Serve the Margaritas in two big tumblers, with a Corona beer on the side. As they sip their Margarita, each individual can include beer to it.

Mixed batch method

1. Inside a mixer, blend the Tequila, Triple Sec, lime juice, simple syrup, orange juice, and a 12-ounce lager. Pour with 4 glasses of ice. Puree the mixture till it is smooth and foamy. Pour into serving glasses and serve.

Nutrition: Calories: 386; Carbohydrates: 51 gm; Protein: 1 gm; Fat: 0 gm; Cholesterol: 55 mg

61. *Spicy Pineapple Habanero Margaritas*

Preparation Time: five mins

Cooking Time: five mins

Total time: ten mins

Servings: six

Ingredients:

- one teacup Tequila Silver
- one teacup Triple Sec
- one teacup fresh-squeezed lime juice
- two and half teacups pineapple juice
- 4 Habanero chilies
- Optional garnishes: salt, limes, Habaneros, pineapple slices

Directions:

1. Dissolve the butter inside a small saucepot at middling temp. Take out the habaneros by cutting them in half. Place chiles in griddle and cook till blistered on both sides. Get out of the fire.

2. In a pitcher, blend the Tequila, Triple Sec, lime juice, and pineapple juice. Stir everything thoroughly.

3. Toss in the blistered Habaneros. Allow them to soak in the Margarita mix for fifteen mins to overnight. The longer they soak in the mixture, the hotter it will get. After fifteen mins, taste the mixture to see how long you want to soak them. When the heat level is to your taste, take out the Habaneros.

4. Pour the Margaritas into glasses with ice when prepared to serve. Garnish with lime wedges, pineapple slices, or more Habaneros if desired.

Nutrition: Calories: 287; Carbohydrates: 31 gm; Protein: 1 gm; Fat: 0 gm; Cholesterol: 65 mg

62. Cranberry Pomegranate Margarita with a Spiced Rim

Preparation Time: five mins

Cooking Time: five mins

Total time: ten mins

Servings: four

Ingredients:

- two teacups cranberry pomegranate juice blend
- two teacups Tequila Blanco
- one teacup freshly squeezed lime juice
- half teacup Triple Sec
- two tbsps coarse sea salt
- one tsp Old El Paso taco seasoning
- two tbsps agave syrup

Directions:

1. One tbsp water and one tbsp agave syrup on a dish to blend, gently mix everything.
2. On a separate dish, blend the salt and Old El Paso taco seasoning.
3. Using the agave syrup, coat the rims of 4-6 glasses. Then, dip the rims in the seasoned salt. Fill the cups halfway with ice.
4. Inside a big ice-filled shaker or pitcher, blend the cranberry pomegranate juice, Tequila, lime juice, and triple sec. Shake or mix prior to pouring into glasses and serving!

Nutrition: Calories: 483; Carbohydrates: 38 gm; Protein: 0 gm; Fat: 0 gm; Cholesterol: 346 mg

63. Peach Milkshake (Copycat Chikk-Fil-a Peach Shake Recipe!)

Preparation Time: five mins

Cooking Time: five mins

Total time: ten mins

Servings: four

Ingredients:

- 6 ripe peaches pitted, skins on
- 7 scoops vanilla ice cream
- three tbsps granulated sugar
- half tsp vanilla extract
- 1 tweak salt
- Optional: whipped cream and Maraschino cherries

Directions:

1. Take out the pits from the peaches, and cut them in half.
2. Blend the peaches, ice cream, sugar, vanilla, and salt inside a big blender.
3. Puree till smooth, covered.

Nutrition: Calories: 397; Carbohydrates: 62 gm; Protein: 7 gm; Fat: 9 gm; Cholesterol: 14 mg

64. Jugo Verde (Green Juice)

Preparation Time: ten mins

Cooking Time: zero mins

Total time: ten mins

Servings: five

Ingredients:

- two teacups orange juice
- one and half teacups fresh pineapple chunks
- 1/2 nopal cactus paddle severed (or substitute 1 celery stalk)
- one big cucumber with peel, cut into chunks
- quarter teacup packed parsley or cilantro

Directions:

1. Inside a mixer, blend the entire components. Include a bit of salt, close the lid tightly, and puree till smooth.
2. When the mixture is green and frothy, serve immediately or strain over a screen to take out the pulp.

Nutrition: Calories: 67; Carbohydrates: 12 gm; Protein: 2 gm; Fat: 2 gm; Cholesterol: 86 mg

65. Perfect Manhattan Recipe

Preparation Time: two mins

Cooking Time: five mins

Total time: seven mins

Servings: one

Ingredients:

- two oz. Bourbon, or Rye whiskey
- 1 oz. Sweet Vermouth, like Antica
- 2 dashes Angostura Bitters
- **Garnishes:** twist lemon rind, orange rind, or a maraschino cherry

Directions:

1. Fill a cocktail shaker halfway with ice for each Manhattan cocktail. Blend the Bourbon, Sweet Vermouth, and bitters in a mixing glass.
2. Using a bar spoon, stir all collectively. Don't jiggle. Then strain into a coupe cocktail glass or a low ball glass filled with ice.
3. Serve with a Maraschino cherry, lemon peel twist, or orange rind twist as a garnish.

Nutrition: Calories: 190; Carbohydrates: 2 gm; Protein: 1 gm; Fat: 16 gm; Cholesterol: 293 mg

66. Frozen Coconut Mojito

Preparation Time: five mins

Cooking Time: five mins

Total time: ten mins

Servings: two

Ingredients:

- 4 oz. coconut cream
- 4 oz. coconut rum

- 2 oz. fresh lime juice
- 8 fresh mint leaves
- four teacups ice

Directions:

1. In a high-powered blender, blend the entire components with four teacups of ice. Pour into glasses after blending, till the mixture is smooth.
2. If desired, garnish with mint and lime slices.

Nutrition: Calories: 386; Carbohydrates: 43 gm; Protein: 1 gm; Fat: 9 gm; Cholesterol: 182 mg

67. Mulled Lemonade Recipe

Preparation Time: twenty mins

Cooking Time: five mins

Total time: twenty-five mins

Servings: eight

Ingredients:

- five teacups water divided
- one teacup granulated sugar
- one teacup fresh lemon juice
- 3 cinnamon sticks
- 6 whole star anise
- 4 slices fresh ginger
- 4 pieces orange peel big
- 20 whole pieces
- 6 cracked green cardamom pods
- half tsp pink peppercorns

Directions:

1. Two teacups of water, brought to a boil mix in the sugar and the entire pieces. Allow the simple syrup to steep for almost twenty mins, covered.
2. Fill a big pitcher halfway with syrup. Then include the rest of the three cups of water and lemon juice. Fill the pitcher halfway with ice and swirl well.

Notes: If you don't want "floaties" in your drinks, drain the spices out of the simple syrup.

Nutrition: Calories: 117; Carbohydrates: 30 gm; Protein: 1 gm; Fat: 1 gm; Cholesterol: 70 mg

68. Cucumber Rose Aperol Spritz

Preparation Time: five mins

Cooking Time: five mins

Total time: ten mins

Servings: one

Ingredients:

- 2 oz. rose-infused Aperol
- 2 oz. sparkling wine such as prosecco
- 2 slices cucumber about an inch dense
- Splash Club Soda

Directions:

1. To make rose-infused Aperol, mix one 750ml bottle Aperol with one ounce dried rose petals (these can be found in the bulk section of most specialty food stores). Shake everything together and set it aside for a few hours or overnight. After straining off the rose petals, the Aperol is ready to use.
2. In a cocktail shaker, blend the rose Aperol and cucumber with ice. Fill a tall collins glass halfway with ice and strain it into it. Pour in the sparkling wine and ice. Garnish with fresh cucumber and a dash of club soda.

Nutrition: Calories: 143; Carbohydrates: 12 gm; Protein: 1 gm; Fat: 1 gm; Cholesterol: 50 mg

69. Pink Grapefruit Margarita

Preparation Time: five mins

Cooking Time: zero mins

Total time: five mins

Servings: two

Ingredients:

- 5 oz. freshly squeezed ruby red grapefruit juice
- 4 oz. white tequila
- 1 1/2 oz. Triple Sec orange liquor
- 1/2 oz. agave syrup + extra for glass rims
- Fresh grapefruit slices for garnish
- Salt for rim

Directions:

1. Put a little quantity of agave syrup on one plate and salt on another. Dip the rims of the glasses first in the syrup, then in the salt. Fill the cups halfway with ice and set them aside.
2. Fill an ice-filled cocktail shaker halfway with ice. Fill the shaker halfway with fresh grapefruit juice, tequila, triple sec, and agave.
3. Cover and vigorously shake for thirty secs. After that, pour into the glasses. Relish with fresh grapefruit slices as a garnish!

Nutrition:

Calories: 251; Carbohydrates: 20 gm; Protein: 1 gm; Fat: 1 gm; Cholesterol: 192 mg

70. Strawberry Margarita Recipe

Preparation Time: ten mins

Cooking Time: zero mins

Total time: ten mins

Servings: two

Ingredients:

- one lb. fresh strawberries, trimmed
- one teacup tequila
- three-quarter teacup fresh lime juice
- two-third teacup strawberry jam
- quarter teacup triple sec
- 10 mint leaves

- three-four teacups ice
- **Optional garnish:** margarita salt, lime slices, extra strawberries

Directions:

1. Prepare a big blender. Include the fresh-cut strawberries, tequila, lime juice, strawberry jam, Triple Sec, mint leaves, and ice to the container.
2. Blend till smooth.
3. **Toppings:** Include additional strawberry jam around the rims of four glasses using a pastry brush. Dip the rims of the glasses in margarita salt.
4. Fill the glass halfway with cold margaritas. Serve with a fresh lime slice and a strawberry on top.

Nutrition: Calories: 391; Carbohydrates: 57 gm; Protein: 1 gm; Fat: 1 gm; Cholesterol: 142 mg

71. **Large-Batch Goombay Smash Caribbean Cocktails**

Preparation Time: five mins

Cooking Time: three mins

Total time: eight mins

Servings: forty

Ingredients:

- fourteen teacups 100% pineapple juice
- two bottles dark Caribbean rum (750 ml each - I used Pusser's)
- 1 bottle coconut rum (750 ml - Cruzan)
- two teacups fresh-squeezed lime juice
- one and half teacups simple syrup
- one teacup orange liqueur (cointreau)
- half tsp bitters, optional
- Fresh pineapple slices for garnish

Directions:

1. If you're creating your simple syrup, mix one teacup granulated sugar and one teacup water. Cook till the sugar melts on the burner. Allow cooling fully.
2. Fill a big beverage dispenser halfway with the entire components. Stir everything together thoroughly. Chill till ready to serve, then top with cut pineapples.
3. Serve with ice.

Nutrition: Calories: 222; Carbohydrates: 22 gm; Protein: 0 gm; Fat: 0 gm; Cholesterol: 11 mg

72. **Healthy Vegan Brownies**

Preparation Time: fifteen mins

Cooking Time: thirty mins

Total time: forty-five mins

Servings: nine

Ingredients:

- 4 tablespoons ground flax
- **two-third teacup** warm water
- one teacup date sugar or coconut sugar

- one teacup cacao powder
- half teacup white whole wheat flour
- ½ tablespoon salt
- one tsp baking powder
- half teacup unsweetened applesauce or pumpkin puree
- one tbsp vanilla extract
- quarter teacup unsweetened almond milk optional

Directions:

1. Warm up the oven to 325 deg.F. In a small dish, blend ground flax and warm water. Allow for a fifteen-min resting period.
2. Inside a medium blending container, blend the dry components (date sugar, cacao powder, white whole wheat flour, baking powder, and salt) while the flax egg is set.
3. In the middle of the dry components, make a well. Blend the wet and dry components (flax egg, applesauce/or pumpkin puree, and vanilla extract). Stir till well mixed. If the batter appears to be too dry, include fourteen teacups of unsweetened almond milk.
4. Pour the batter into an eight-inch square baking dish lined with parchment paper. Distribute evenly.
5. Keep thirty to thirty-five mins in the oven, or till a toothpick inserted in the middle comes out clean. Allow cooling fully in the pan prior to removing and cutting into squares.

Nutrition: Calories: 126; Carbohydrates: 28 gm; Protein: 3 gm; Fat: 1 gm; Cholesterol: 172 mg

73. **Green Chicken Soup**

Preparation Time: fifteen mins

Cooking Time: twenty-five mins

Total time: forty mins

Servings: twelve

Ingredients:

- 2/4 chicken broth or stock
- one and half lbs. boneless, skinless chicken breast
- two celery stalks, severed
- two teacups green beans, cut into one inch pieces
- one and half teacups peas, fresh or frozen
- two teacups asparagus, cut into one inch pieces, tops, and middles (avoid tough ends)
- one teacup cubed green onions
- 4-6 garlic pieces, crushed
- two teacups fresh spinach leaves, severed and packed
- 1 bunch watercress, severed with big stems taken out
- half teacup fresh parsley leaves, severed
- one-third teacup fresh basil leaves, severed
- one tsp salt

Directions:

1. Inside a big saucepan, boil the chicken broth at medium-high temp. Bring the chicken breasts to a simmer in the sauce.

2. Blend the celery, green beans, peas, asparagus, onions, garlic, and salt inside a blending container. Simmer for five-ten mins, or till the vegetables are soft, then take out from the heat.

3. Take out the chicken breasts and shred or cut them into bite-sized pieces with two forks. Back to the pot.

4. Blend the spinach, watercress, parsley, and basil inside a blending container. Season with salt as required.

Nutrition: Calories: 105; Carbohydrates: 7 gm; Protein: 15 gm; Fat: 2 gm; Cholesterol: 134 mg

74. Green Risotto Recipe

Preparation Time: ten mins

Cooking Time: forty mins

Total time: fifty mins

Servings: eight

Ingredients:

- two teacups arborio rice
- three tbsps butter
- three tbsps olive oil
- 6 scallions, greens, and whites severed
- two and half teacups fresh packed spinach leaves
- one teacup packed fresh parsley
- 12 fresh basil leaves
- 3 garlic pieces
- six teacups chicken broth, room temp. (vegetable broth for vegetarians)
- one teacup white wine
- one teacup shredded Parmesan cheese
- Salt

Directions:

1. Inside a mixer, blend spinach, parsley, basil, and garlic. Include four teacups broth and purée till entirely smooth.

2. Inside a big sauté pan, blend the butter and oil. In a medium saucepan at middling temp., melt the butter. Include the scallions once the butter has melted and cooked for two mins. After adding the rice, cook for an extra two mins. Then stir in the wine, one and half tsps of salt, and half tsp ground.

3. Simmer, occasionally stirring, till the wine has been absorbed. Start with the two teacups of liquid that was not put into the blender and include one cup of broth at a time to the rice. Stir the rice after each addition of liquid and let it boil till the broth is absorbed prior to adding more. Ensure that the entire green herb broth is included in the blender. This procedure will take approximately twenty-five mins.

4. Stir in the grated parmesan cheese after you've poured the rest of the green liquid and the rice is cooked but still firm. Turn off the heat prior to the last round of stock has been entirely absorbed, leaving the risotto a bit soupy. As it cools, it will stiffen up. Season as required with salt and serve warm.

Nutrition:

Calories: 283; Carbohydrates: 36 gm; Protein: 1 gm; Fat: 1 gm; Cholesterol: 53 mg

Snacks

75. Mango Pudding (Dairy-Free!) Recipe

Preparation Time: fifteen mins

Cooking Time: five mins

Total time: twenty mins

Servings: eleven

Ingredients:

- two teacups mango puree from two big juicy mangos
- 13.5 oz. can unsweetened coconut milk
- one teacup hot water
- one teacup granulated sugar
- 5 teaspoons unflavored gelatin powder measured from 2 packets
- one tsp vanilla extract
- Pinch salt

Directions:

1. Place a big liquid measuring cup on the table. Blend the boiling water, sugar, gelatin, and salt inside a blending container. Allow the mixture to rest for five mins after thoroughly stirring.

2. Meanwhile, peel and chop the mangoes into big bits. Take out the pits and peels. Inside a mixer, blend the mango pieces. Puree till smooth, then measure out two teacups. (if necessary, scoop some out of the mixer.)

3. Blend in the coconut milk and vanilla extract. Blend till smooth. Then include the gelatin mixture to the blender and blend till smooth. Puree one more till smooth.

4. Fill tiny 4-ounce serving glasses halfway with mango pudding. To set, cover and put in the fridge the cups for three-four hrs. Garnish with mint and serve chilled. Garnish with toasted coconut, lime zest, or severed cashews if desired.

Note: you may alternatively use frozen mango pieces that have been thawed. Store in the fridge, covered, for up to 5 days.

Nutrition: Calories: 174; Carbohydrates: 26 gm; Protein: 18 gm; Fat: 8 gm; Cholesterol: 281 mg

76. Banana Oatmeal Chocolate Chip Cookies (Healthy!)

Preparation Time: fifteen mins

Cooking Time: twelve mins

Total time: twenty-seven mins

Servings: eighteen

Ingredients:

- two teacups quick oats
- half teacup almond flour
- 3 big brown bananas mashed (about one teacup)
- half teacup light brown sugar or palm sugar
- one big egg
- two tsps baking powder
- one tsp vanilla extract
- quarter tsp salt
- quarter teacups dark chocolate chips

Directions:

1. Warm up the oven to 350 deg.F. 2 big baking sheets, lined with parchment paper.
2. Blend the oats, almond flour, mashed bananas, brown sugar, egg, baking powder, vanilla extract, and salt in an electric stand mixer container. Beat the mixture till it is smooth and uniform.
3. Then, with the mixer on low, fold in half of the chocolate chips.
4. To distribute the cookies onto the baking pans, use a 1.5 tablespoon cookie scoop. Set them apart by 2 inches.
5. Place 4-5 chocolate chips on top of each cookie, flattening the dough balls slightly.
6. Bake for twelve mins or till the edges are firm. Cool for five mins on the cookie sheets prior to transferring.

Nutrition: Calories: 192; Carbohydrates: 24 gm; Protein: 51 gm; Fat: 9 gm; Cholesterol: 261 mg

77. Larabar Snack Bar

Preparation Time: five mins

Cooking Time: five mins

Total time: ten mins

Servings: twelve

Ingredients:

- two teacups raw almonds
- three-quarter teacup pitted dates packed
- one teacup dried unsweetened apples
- quarter teacup raisins packed
- half tsp cinnamon
- quarter tsp sea salt

Directions:

1. Inside a blending container, blend the entire components and process till finely severed and sticky.
2. Line an eight inch baking dish with wax paper, leaving enough to hang over the sides to cover the mixture. Fill the dish halfway with the mixture and top with

wax paper. Press or roll out the components till it is smooth.

3. Take out the wax paper and bars from the pan and cut them into 12 equal bars. Wrap each piece in wax paper and store it in a sealed container.

Nutrition: Calories: 153; Carbohydrates: 17 gm; Protein: 17 gm; Fat: 27 gm; Cholesterol: 89 mg

78. Kulfi Indian Ice Cream

Preparation Time: ten mins

Cooking Time: one hundred and sixty mins

Total time: one hundred and seventy mins

Servings: sixteen

Ingredients:

- two teacups heavy cream
- 14 oz. can sweeten condensed milk
- 2 teaspoon ground cardamom
- one tsp vanilla extract
- half teacup severed pistachios
- A tweak saffron + one tbsp. warm water

Directions:

1. In a small dish, blend one tbsp hot tap water. Allow a tweak of saffron to soak to absorb its color and taste.
2. Meanwhile, prepare an electric mixer fitted with a whip attachment. Pour in the heavy cream, cardamom powder, and vanilla essence. Whip the mixture at high speed till firm peaks form.
3. Using a rubber spatula, scrape the container. Then include the saffron and water and mix well.
4. Fold in the sweetened condensed milk using a spatula. Fold in the severed pistachios after the mixture is smooth and uniform.
5. Insert the kulfi in a sealed container and freeze it, or spoon it into tiny cups for popsicles and place a popsicle stick in the center of each one.
6. Freeze for a minimum of three hrs.

Nutrition: Calories: 200; Carbohydrates: 16 gm; Protein: 14 gm; Fat: 18 gm; Cholesterol: 44 mg

79. Easy No-Bake Key Lime Pie Recipe

Preparation Time: twenty mins

Cooking Time: two hundred and forty mins

Total time: two hundred and sixty mins

Servings: eight

Ingredients:

For the graham cracker crust:

- 12 whole graham crackers crushed (about one and half teacups)
- 6 tablespoons melted butter
- quarter teacup granulated sugar
- quarter tsp salt

For the key lime pie filling:

- 8-oz. cream cheese softened
- 14-oz. sweetened condensed milk
- half teacup key lime juice
- 3-5 drops lime green food coloring if desired
- 8-oz. cool whip
- Lime zest for garnish

Directions:

1. Prepare a 9-inch pie pan as well as a food processor. Inside a blending container, blend the graham crackers. Close the lid and pulse into a fine crumb. After that, stir in the melted butter, sugar, and salt. To mix, pulse the components together.

2. Fill the pie pan halfway with the graham cracker crumble. Press it into an equal layer over the bottom and up the edges of the pan with your hands. Keep refrigerated till ready to use.

3. Wipe the food processor container clean. Then blend the cream cheese, sweetened condensed milk, and lime juice inside a blending container. Blend till smooth. (if wanted, include food coloring here.)

4. Take the food processor blade out of the machine. Scoop the cool whip into the lime mixture and stir well. Wrap the cool whip into the mixture with a spatula till entirely smooth.

5. Fill the pie crust with the filling. Then, store the mixture in the freezer for almost four hrs, undisturbed.

6. If preferred, top with fresh lime zest when ready to serve. While still frozen, cut into pieces. Allow each piece to remain at room temp. for ten mins prior to serving somewhat softened.

Nutrition: Calories: 451; Carbohydrates: 60 gm; Protein: 63 gm; Fat: 28 gm; Cholesterol: 59 mg

80. Lemon Cheesecake Recipe (Limoncello Cake!)

Preparation Time: twenty mins

Cooking Time: sixty mins

Total time: eighty mins

Servings: sixteen

Ingredients:

For the Biscoff crust:

- 8.8 oz. Biscoff cookies, 1 package
- half teacup granulated sugar
- half tsp salt
- half teacup unsalted butter, melted

For the limoncello cheesecake filling:

- 24 oz. cream cheese, softened
- four big eggs
- three-quarter teacup granulated sugar
- one big lemon, zested and juiced (quarter teacup juice)
- quarter teacup limoncello liqueur

- half tsp vanilla extract
- half tsp salt

For the sour cream topping

- 16 oz. sour cream
- quarter teacup granulated sugar
- three tbsps limoncello liqueur

Directions:

1. Warm up the oven to 350 deg.F. Put one oven rack in the center and one at the bottom of the oven. To catch any spillage, use a big rimmed baking sheet on the bottom rack. Warm up the oven to 350 deg.F. Line the bottom of a nine and half inch springform pan with parchment paper. Then, securely tighten the ring around the bottom. (If desired, trim the paper edges.)

2. To make the crust: inside a blending container, blend the Biscoff cookies, sugar, and salt. Pulse the cookies till they are finely ground. After that, include the dissolved butter and pulse to the mix. Fill the prepared pan halfway with the crust mixture. With your hands, press the crumbs all over the bottom of the pan and approximately two-thirds of the way up the edges. Ten mins in the oven.

3. Meanwhile, prepare the limoncello cheesecake filling by placing the cream cheese in the container of an electric mixer. Two mins on high to soften and fluff the cream cheese. Include the eggs one at a time, delaying adding another till the preceding egg is thoroughly mixed in. Using a spatula, scrape the container. Then mix in the other components till fully smooth—bake for forty-five mins after pouring the filling into the crust.

4. To make the sour cream topping, blend the sour cream, sugar, and limoncello in a medium mixing container and whisk till smooth. Once the cheesecake has baked and is nearly set in the center, pour the sour cream filling over the top and return to the oven for ten-twelve mins.

5. Leave for one hr on the counter to cool the cheesecake. Then put in the fridge for almost three hrs to cool. Take out the ring from the springform pan and place the cheesecake on a cake plate. Cut into slices and serve chilled.

Nutrition: Calories: 386; Carbohydrates: 35 gm; Protein: 22 gm; Fat: 17 gm; Cholesterol: 108 mg

81. Dark Chocolate with Pomegranate Seeds

Preparation Time: ten mins

Cooking Time: two-three mins

Servings: three

Ingredients:

- 150 gm dark chocolate (almost 70% cocoa)
- 120 gm pomegranate seeds (from 1 pomegranate)
- one tsp sea salt

Directions:

1. Scatter a layer of pomegranate seeds in a muffin tin (or muffin paper).
2. Melt the chocolate in the microwave.
3. Pour the chocolate into a bag, then cut a tiny hole so that it can be spread over the seeds. Include a layer of seeds and another of chocolate.
4. Spray with a tweak of salt and chill in the fridge till the mixture is hard.
5. Relish cold.

Nutrition: Calories: 82; Carbs: 19 gm; Protein: 1.9 gm; Fat: 0.2 gm; Sugar: 3.9 gm; Sodium: 37 mg; Fiber: 3.7 gm

82. Covered Bananas

Preparation Time: ten mins

Cooking Time: zero mins

Servings: three

Ingredients:

- 3 bananas
- one tbsp oat bran
- two tbsps cashew or almond butter
- one tbsp honey
- one tsp chia seeds
- one tsp cinnamon

Directions:

1. Mix the oat bran, seeds, and cinnamon in a shallow container.
2. Mix the nut butter with honey.
3. Coat the bananas with nut butter and then include to the dry mixture so that they are coated on both sides.

Nutrition: Calories: 11; Carbs: 3 gm; Protein: 0 gm; Fat: 0 gm; Sugar: 2.9 gm; Sodium: 0 mg; Fiber: 0.1 gm

83. Hummus with Tahini and Turmeric

Preparation Time: ten mins

Cooking Time: zero mins

Servings: four

Ingredients:

- two cans chickpeas, drained
- 50 ml lemon juice
- 60 ml tahini
- 1 garlic piece, crushed
- two tbsps extra-virgin olive oil
- half tbsp turmeric powder
- half tsp sea salt

Directions:

1. Mix the tahini and lemon juice with olive oil, garlic, turmeric, and salt for around thirty secs using a hand blender or kitchen utensil.
2. Include the chickpeas and puree, making sure that no chickpeas remain unmixed on the sides. Pound till a uniform mixture is obtained.

3. Garnish with paprika powder and relish with any snacks, such as vegetable sticks.

Nutrition: Calories: 33 gm; Carbs: 8.1 gm; Protein: 0.2 gm; Fat: 0.1 gm; Sugar: 7.6 gm; Sodium: 130 mg; Fiber: 0.1 gm

84. Pineapple Orange Creamsicle

Preparation Time: ten mins

Cooking Time: twelve mins

Total time: twenty-two mins

Servings: ten

Ingredients:

- two teacups orange-pineapple juice
- one teacup heavy cream
- half teacup granulated sugar
- two tsps vanilla extract

Directions:

1. In a microwave-safe container, blend half teacup juice and 1/2 sugar. Warm the juice for 1-two mins or till the sugar melts. Then include the rest of the juice and whisk to blend.
2. Pour the heavy cream, vanilla extract, and 1 quarter teacup of the sweetened juice into a separate dish (or measuring pitcher). Stir everything together thoroughly. Then divide the mixture evenly among ten regular popsicle molds.
3. For one hr, place the popsicles in the freezer. Then, drizzle the rest of the juice over the tops of each popsicle and insert wooden popsicle sticks. Freeze for almost three hrs more.

Nutrition: Calories: 145; Carbohydrates: 15 gm; Protein: 17 gm; Fat: 8 gm; Cholesterol: 76 mg

85. Easy Peach Cobbler Recipe with Bisquick

Preparation Time: ten mins

Cooking Time: sixty mins

Total time: seventy mins

Servings: seven

Ingredients:

- 48 oz. fresh or frozen sliced peaches six and half teacups, with or without peels
- two teacups granulated sugar
- half tsp of pumpkin pie spice or apple pie spice blend
- 2 Cups Bisquick baking mix
- one teacup whole milk
- one teacup melted butter

Directions:

1. Warm up the oven to 350 deg.F. Prepare a nine by thirteen inch baking dish and a big mixing basin.
2. If you are using fresh peaches, cut them into wedges and take out the pits. Fill the baking dish halfway with fresh (or frozen) peach slices. Then, over the peaches, include one teacup sugar and the pumpkin pie spice.

Toss the peach to coat it, then spread it out in an equal layer.

3. Blend the rest of the one teacup sugar, Bisquick, and milk in a mixing basin. Whisk everything together well. Then include the melted butter and stir till blended.

4. Pour the batter over the peaches in an equal layer. Bake for fifty-five to sixty mins, depending on the size of the baking dish.

5. After forty mins, check on the cobbler. If the top begins to darken, loosely cover with foil and continue baking.

6. Allow almost fifteen mins for the cobbler to cool prior to serving. Serve in dishes with vanilla ice cream or whipped cream.

Notes: you don't like peaches? Replace with nectarines, plums, pitted cherries.

How to keep leftovers: once the cobbler has entirely cooled, cover it in plastic wrap or move it to a container with a lid. The fruit cobbler may be stored in the fridge for up to 4-5 days.

To put on ice: cook according to the recipe in a freezer-safe baking dish, cool, and cover the entire dish in plastic wrap. Wrap in tin foil and place in the freezer for up to 3 months. Unwrap and bake in a 350 deg.F oven for forty-fifty mins, or till boiling.

Nutrition: Calories: 420; Carbohydrates: 59 gm; Protein: 11 gm; Fat: 20 gm; Cholesterol: 172 mg

86. Healthy 5-Minute Strawberry Pineapple Sherbet

Preparation Time: five mins

Cooking Time: five mins

Total time: ten mins

Servings: sixteen

Ingredients:

- one lb. frozen strawberries
- one lb. has frozen pineapple chunks
- half teacup plain Greek yogurt
- half teacup honey or palm syrup
- two tsps vanilla extract
- A tweak salt

Directions:

1. Inside a big food mixer, blend the entire components. Pulse the frozen fruit to break it up. Then purée till entirely smooth.

2. Serve immediately as soft serve, or freeze in a sealed container. Thaw for fifteen mins prior to scooping and serving if frozen.

Notes: This sherbet has a distinct honey taste. If you dislike the flavor of honey, use palm syrup.

Nutrition: Calories: 70; Carbohydrates: 16 gm; Protein: 2 gm; Fat: 1 gm; Cholesterol: 1 mg

87. Best Coconut Milk Ice Cream (Dairy-Free!)

Preparation Time: three mins

Cooking Time: thirty mins

Total time: thirty-three mins

Servings: sixteen

Ingredients:

- 27-oz. canned full-fat unsweetened coconut milk 2 cans
- 13.6-oz. can coconut cream
- one teacup granulated sugar
- two tsps of vanilla extract or vanilla bean paste
- quarter tsp salt

Directions:

1. After making this ice cream numerous times, I learned that it does not always need to be heated/cooked prior to churning... This saves a huge amount of time. (This depends on the kind of coconut milk/cream and the kind of blender you use.) Put the entire components inside a blender and purée till smooth to see whether your ice cream has to be cooked. If the coconut ice cream mixture is smooth and free of clumps, you may churn it without heating.

2. Heat and stir: if there are any pieces of coconut cream in the recipe, they will freeze as hard waxy clumps in the ice cream. In this scenario, cook the mixture at middling temp. till smooth, stirring often. Before churning, chill and cool to almost room temp.. If you don't want to "test" the no-heat approach, simply blend all components in a saucepot and cook at middling temp. till smooth, allowing the coconut clumps and sugar to dissolve. Then take a break.

3. Set out a 1.5-2 quart ice cream machine after the ice cream mixture has cooled. Turn on the machine and place the frozen container inside. Fill the machine halfway with the extremely smooth ice cream mixture. Cook for twenty to twenty-five mins, or till the mixture is dense, hard, and smooth.

4. Serve immediately, or transfer to a sealed container and freeze till ready to use.

Nutrition: Calories: 224; Carbohydrates: 16 gm; Protein: 2 gm; Fat: 19 gm; Cholesterol: 27 mg

88. Lemon Crinkle Cookies Recipe

Preparation Time: fifteen mins

Cooking Time: ten mins

Total time: twenty-five mins

Servings: forty-five

Ingredients:

- one teacup unsalted butter, softened (2 sticks)
- three-quarter teacups granulated sugar
- four big eggs
- two tbsps fresh lemon juice

- two tbsps lemon zest
- one tsp vanilla extract
- one teacup all-purpose flour (stir, spoon into the cup, and level)
- 2 teaspoon baking powder
- half tsp salt
- quarter tsp baking soda
- 2-5 drops yellow food coloring (optional)
- two teacups powdered sugar

Directions:

1. In the container of an electric stand mixer, blend the butter and granulated sugar. Cream the butter and sugar together on high for three-five mins, or till light and creamy. Using a rubber spatula, scrape the container.
2. Mix in the eggs, lemon juice, lemon zest, and vanilla extract at low speed. Scrape the container once more. Mix in one teacup of flour, baking powder, salt, baking soda, and food coloring on low. Once mixed, gently fold in the rest of the two teacups of flour till smooth.
3. Refrigerate the dough for almost thirty mins, covered. Warm up the oven to 375 deg.F. Set aside several baking sheets lined with parchment paper.
4. Set out a small dish of powdered sugar once the dough has cooled. To separate the dough into balls, use a one tbsp cookie scoop. Roll each ball in powdered sugar, then place 2 inches apart on baking pans.
5. For nine-ten mins, or till the sides are golden brown and the middle appears slightly underbaked. Allow them to cool on the baking pans so that the centers continue to bake as they cool.

Note: Storage suggestions: Store the cookies in a sealed jar at room temp. Consume within 7-10 days.

Citrus substitutions: in place of the lemon, you can use lime or orange juice and zest. You may also blend lemon and lime for a unique taste combination!

Nutrition: Calories: 111; Carbohydrates: 16 gm; Protein: 29 gm; Fat: 18 gm; Cholesterol: 63 mg

The Best No-Bake Chocolate Lasagna

Preparation Time: twenty mins

Cooking Time: one hundred and twenty mins

Total time: one hundred and forty mins

Servings: twelve

Ingredients:

Oreo layer

- 40 oreo cookies
- 7 tablespoons melted butter

Cream cheese layer

- eight oz. cream cheese, softened
- three tbsps granulated sugar
- two tbsps milk
- 16 oz. cool whip, reserve half for later

Chocolate pudding layer:

- 7.8 oz. instant chocolate pudding mix two small boxes
- two and three-quarter teacups of milk
- two tsps instant coffee granules

Whipped topping layer:

- Remaining cool whip
- two teacups mini chocolate chips or half teacup chocolate shavings

Directions:

1. Set up a big food processor to make the oreo crust. Inside a blending dish, blend the oreo cookies. Cover and pulse till tiny crumbs form. Then, pulse in the melted butter to coat. * If you don't have a food processor, you may smash the cookies with a rolling pin in a zip bag. Then, for the rest of the processes, use a mixer.
2. Fill a nine by thirteen inch baking dish halfway with oreo crumbs. Chill after pressing into a uniform layer.
3. A layer of cream cheese: next, rinse off the food processor container. Blend the cream cheese, sugar, and milk inside a blending container. Blend till smooth. Then, using a knife, spoon half (8 oz.) of the cool whip into the cream cheese. Fold the mixture with a spatula till it is smooth. Spread the mixture evenly over the crust in the baking dish. Chill.
4. Rinse the food processor container once more for the chocolate pudding layer. Blend the chocolate pudding powder, milk, and instant coffee inside a blending container. Puree till smooth, covered. In the baking dish, evenly distribute the components.
5. Toppings: top the chocolate pudding with the rest of the 8 oz. of cool whip. Then, over the top, sprinkle with tiny chocolate chips or chocolate shavings.
6. Put in the fridge for almost four hrs, covered. Freeze for two-three hrs for optimum cutting results, then cut and serve. Allow ten-fifteen mins for the frozen plated pieces to come to room temp. prior to serving.

Note: this is a fantastic make-ahead dessert that can be made 4-5 days ahead of time and stored in the freezer for up to 3 months.

Nutrition: Calories: 533; Carbohydrates: 72 gm; Protein: 16 gm; Fat: 8 gm; Cholesterol: 42 mg

89. **Healthy Watermelon Smoothie Recipe Easiest**

Preparation Time: three mins

Cooking Time: three mins

Total time: six mins

Servings: four

Ingredients:

- four teacups fresh ripe watermelon cubes from a less melon

- two teacups strawberry yogurt regular or a dairy-free variety
- four teacups ice
- one-two tbsps granulated sugar optional (only needed if the watermelon isn't very sweet.)

Directions:

1. Inside a mixer, blend the watermelon cubes and yogurt. Puree till smooth, covered. Taste to see if more sugar is required.
2. Pour in the ice cubes (and sugar if desired). After that, cover and purée till smooth.
3. Serve immediately.

Note: Garnish with cubes or slices of watermelon or cut strawberries.

Nutrition: Calories: 120; Carbohydrates: 27 gm; Protein: 27 gm; Fat: 19 gm; Cholesterol: 47 mg

90. Watermelon

When looking for the right watermelon, keep in mind the following characteristics: stripes are well defined, with noticeable color differences between the green and yellow lines. A huge yellow patch on the bottom indicates that the watermelon has been ripening on the vine in the field for some time and was not harvested too early.

Preparation Time: five mins

Cooking Time: five mins

Total time: ten mins

Servings: four

Ingredients:

- Whole watermelon

Directions:

1. Take out the melon's short (stem) ends. Then, from stem end to stem end, cut the watermelon into quarters.
2. Start at the top of the fruit and cut straight down to the rind in twelve to one inch portions for slices.
3. Then, on each side, cut along the rind's edge, deep into the watermelon to take out the slices from the rind.
4. To make cubes, cut 1 inch deep into each flat side of the watermelon. Make sure to do this on both sides.
5. Then, starting at the top, cut down in one inch chunks.
6. Finally, cut along the rind's edge on both sides to release the rind cubes.

Nutrition: Calories: 55; Carbohydrates: 10 gm; Protein: 13 gm; Fat: 1 gm; Cholesterol: 10 mg

91. Best Orange Julius

Preparation Time: five mins

Cooking Time: five mins

Total time: ten mins

Servings: three

Ingredients:

- 6-oz. orange juice concentrate, half a can
- one teacup milk 2% or whole
- half teacup water
- one-third teacup granulated sugar
- three tbsps egg white
- two tsps vanilla extract
- three-quarter teacups ice cubes

Directions:

1. Put the entire components in the blender.
2. Puree till smooth.

Note: This orange Julius copy recipe includes 2 big (20 oz. each) or 4 mini (10 oz.) Beverages. Do you want to make a strawberry or pineapple orange Julius? Substitute 8 oz. frozen strawberries or frozen pineapple pieces for the orange juice concentrate.

Nutrition: Calories: 179; Carbohydrates: 36 gm; Protein: 4 gm; Fat: 1 gm; Cholesterol: 6 mg

Dinner

92. Chicken Bone Broth

Preparation Time: ten mins

Cooking Time: ninety mins

Servings: eight

Ingredients:

- three-four lbs. bones (from 1 chicken)
- four teacups water
- two big carrots, cut into chunks
- two big celery stalks
- one big onion
- two teacups fresh rosemary sprigs
- 3 fresh thyme sprigs
- two tbsps apple cider vinegar
- one tsp Kosher salt

Directions:

1. Put the entire components in your pot and allow to sit for thirty mins.
2. Pressure cook and adjust the time to ninety mins.
3. Set the release naturally till the float valve drops and then unlock the lid.
4. Strain the broth and transfer it into a storage container. The broth can be refrigerated for 3-5 days or frozen for up to 6 months.

Nutrition: Calories: 140; Carbs: 0.6 gm; Protein: 25 gm; Fat: 2.6 gm; Sugar: 0.1 gm; Sodium: 73 mg; Fiber: 0.1 gm

93. Homemade Beef Stock

Preparation Time: ten mins

Cooking Time: two-twelve hrs

Servings: six

Ingredients:

- two lbs. beef bones (preferably with marrow)
- 5 celery stalks, severed
- 4 carrots, severed
- 1 white or Spanish onion, severed
- two garlic pieces, crushed
- two bay leaves
- one tsp dried thyme
- one tsp dried sage
- one tsp black peppercorns
- Salt

Directions:

1. Warm up the oven to 425 **deg.F.**
2. On a baking sheet, spread out the beef bones, celery, carrots, onion, garlic, and bay leaves. Spray the thyme, sage, and peppercorns over the top.
3. Roast till the vegetables and bones have a rich brown color.
4. Transfer the roasted bones and vegetables to a big stockpot. Cover with water and slowly bring to a boil over high heat.
5. Set the heat to medium-low for almost two hrs and up to twelve hrs.
6. Pour the mixture through a fine-mesh strainer into a big container.
7. Taste and season with salt. Serve warm.

Nutrition: Calories: 37; Fat: 1 gm; Carbs: 3 gm; Fiber: 0 gm; Protein: 4 gm; Sodium: 58 mg

94. **Three-Ingredient Sugar-Free Gelatin**

Preparation Time: five mins

Cooking Time: zero mins

Servings: six-eight

Ingredients:

- quarter teacup room temp. water
- quarter teacup hot water
- one tbsp gelatin
- one teacup orange juice, unsweetened

Directions:

1. Blend your gelatin and room temp. water, stirring till fully melted.
2. Stir in hot water then leave to rest for around two mins.
3. Include in the juice and stir till blended.
4. Transfer to serving size containers then place on a tray in the fridge to set for around four hrs.
5. Relish!

Nutrition: Calories: 17; Fat: 0 gm; Carbs: 4 gm; Fiber: 0 gm; Protein: 0 gm

95. **Cranberry-Kombucha Jell-O**

Preparation Time: five mins

Cooking Time: zero mins

Servings: six

Ingredients:

- quarter teacup room temp. water
- quarter teacup hot water
- one tbsp gelatin
- one teacup cranberry kombucha, unsweetened

Directions:

1. Blend your gelatin and room temp. water, stirring till fully melted.
2. Stir in hot water then leave to rest for around two mins.
3. Include in the kombucha and stir till blended.
4. Transfer to serving size containers then place on a tray in the fridge to set for around four hrs.
5. Relish!

Nutrition: Calories: 13; Fat: 0 gm; Carbs: 1 gm; Fiber: 0 gm; Protein: 0 gm

96. **Strawberry Gummies**

Preparation Time: five mins

Cooking Time: five mins

Servings: 20-40 mini gummies

Ingredients:

- one teacup strawberries, hulled and severed
- three-quarter teacup water
- two tbsps gelatin

Directions:

1. Bring your water and berries to a boil on high heat. Detach from the heat when the mixture begins to boil.
2. Transfer to the blender and pulse. Include in your gelatin then blend once more.
3. Pour the mixture into a silicone gummy mold.
4. Place on a tray in the fridge to set for around four hrs.
5. Relish!

Nutrition: Calories: 3; Fat: 0 gm; Carbs: 0 gm; Fiber: 0 gm; Protein: 0 gm

97. **Fruity Jell-O Stars**

Preparation Time: fifteen mins

Cooking Time: five mins

Servings: four

Ingredients:

- one tbsp gelatin, powdered
- three-quarter teacup boiling water
- three and half teacups fruit
- one tbsp honey
- one tsp lemon juice

Directions:

1. Attach all your components into a blender and pulse.
2. Include in the gelatin then blend once more.

3. Pour the mixture into a silicone gummy mold.
4. Place on a tray in the fridge to set for around four hrs.
5. Relish!

Nutrition: Calories: 2; Fat: 14 gm; Carbs: 0 gm; Fiber: 1 gm; Protein: 0 gm

98. Sugar-Free Cinnamon Jelly

Preparation Time: five mins

Cooking Time: zero mins

Servings: two

Ingredients:

- one teacup hot cinnamon tea
- one teacup room temp. water
- two tsps gelatin
- one-third teacup sweetener

Directions:

1. Blend your gelatin and room temp. water, stirring till fully melted.
2. Stir in hot tea then leave to rest for around two mins.
3. Include in the sweetener and stir till blended.
4. Transfer to serving size containers then place on a tray in the fridge to set for around four hrs.
5. Relish!

Nutrition: Calories: 35; Fat: 0 gm; Carbs: 17 gm; Fiber: 0 gm; Protein: 0 gm

99. Homey Clear Chicken Broth

Preparation Time: ten mins

Cooking Time: two-twelve hrs

Servings: six teacups

Ingredients:

- two lbs. chicken neck
- two celery ribs with leaves, cut into chunks
- two medium carrots, cut into chunks
- two medium onions, quartered
- two bay leaves
- 2 quarts cold water
- Salt

Directions:

1. Transfer the bones and vegetables to your stockpot. Top with sufficient water to cover then allow to slowly come to a boil on high heat.
2. Switch to low heat and simmer for almost two hrs and up to twelve hrs.
3. Set and pour the mixture through a fine-mesh strainer into a big container.
4. Taste and season with salt.
5. Serve warm.

Nutrition: Calories: 245; Fat: 14 gm; Carbs: 8 gm; Fiber: 2 gm; Protein: 21 gm

100. Oxtail Bone Broth

Preparation Time: fifteen mins

Cooking Time: twelve hrs

Servings: eight teacups

Ingredients:

- two lbs. Oxtail
- 1 onion, severed in quarters
- two celery stalks, severed in half
- 2 carrots, severed in half
- 3 whole garlic pieces
- two bay leaves
- one tbsp salt
- Filtered water (enough to cover bones)

Directions:

1. Transfer the bones and vegetables to your stockpot. Top with sufficient water to cover then allow to slowly come to a boil on high heat.
2. Switch to low heat and simmer for almost two hrs and up to twelve hrs.
3. Set and pour the mixture through a fine-mesh strainer into a big container.
4. Taste and season with salt.
5. Serve warm.

Nutrition: Calories: 576; Fat: 48 gm; Carbs: 48 gm; Fiber: 0 gm; Protein: 24 gm

101. Chicken Bone Broth with Ginger and Lemon

Preparation Time: ten mins

Cooking Time: ninety mins

Servings: eight

Ingredients:

- three-four lbs. bones (from 1 chicken)
- eight teacups water
- two big carrots, cut into chunks
- two big celery stalks
- one big onion
- 3 fresh rosemary sprigs
- 3 fresh thyme sprigs
- two tbsps apple cider vinegar
- one tsp Kosher salt
- 1 (1/2 inches) piece fresh ginger, sliced (peeling not necessary)
- one big lemon, cut into quarters

Directions:

1. Put the entire components in your pot and allow to sit for thirty mins.
2. Pressure cook and adjust the time to 9zero mins.
3. Set the broth using a fine-mesh strainer and transfer it into a storage container.

4. Can be refrigerated for 5 days or frozen for 6 months.

Nutrition: Calories: 44; Fat: 1 gm; Protein: 7 gm; Sodium: 312 mg; Fiber: 0 gm; Carbs: 0 gm; Sugar: 0 gm

102. Vegetable Stock

Preparation Time: ten mins

Cooking Time: forty mins

Servings: eight

Ingredients:

- two big carrots
- one big onion
- two big celery stalks
- 8 oz. white mushrooms
- 5 whole garlic pieces
- two teacups parsley leaves
- two bay leaves
- two tsps whole black peppercorns
- two tsps kosher salt
- 10 cups water

Directions:

1. Place the entire components in your pot. Secure the lid.
2. Pressure cook and adjust the time to forty mins.
3. Set the broth using a fine-mesh strainer and transfer it into a storage container.

Nutrition: Calories: 9; Fat: 0 gm; Protein: 0 gm; Sodium: 585 mg; Fiber: 0 gm; Carbs: 2 gm; Sugar: 1 gm

103. Chicken Vegetable Soup

Preparation Time: twenty-three mins

Cooking Time: fifteen mins

Servings: eight

Ingredients:

- two tbsps avocado oil
- 1 small yellow onion, skinned and severed
- two big carrots, skinned and severed
- two big stalks celery, ends taken out and sliced
- 3 garlic pieces, crushed
- one tsp dried thyme
- one tsp salt
- eight teacups chicken stock
- 3 boneless, skinless, frozen chicken breasts

Directions:

1. Heat the oil for one min. Include the onion, carrots, and celery and sauté for eight mins.
2. Include the garlic, thyme, and salt then sauté for an extra thirty secs. Press the Cancel button.
3. Include the stock and frozen chicken breasts to the pot. Secure the lid.
4. Pressure cook and adjust the time to six mins.

5. Allow cooling into bowls to serve.

Nutrition: Calories: 209; Fat: 7 gm; Protein: 21 gm; Sodium: 687 mg; Fiber: 1 gm; Carbs: 12 gm; Sugar: 5 gm

104. Carrot Ginger Soup

Preparation Time: twenty mins

Cooking Time: twenty-one mins

Servings: four

Ingredients:

- one tbsp avocado oil
- one big yellow onion, skinned and severed
- one lb. carrots, skinned and severed
- one tbsp fresh ginger, skinned and crushed
- one and half tsps salt
- three teacups vegetable broth

Directions:

1. Include the oil to the inner pot, allowing it to heat for one min.
2. Attach the onion, carrots, ginger, and salt then sauté for five mins. Press the Cancel button.
3. Include the broth and secure the lid. Adjust the time to fifteen mins.
4. Allow the soup to cool a couple of mins and then transfer it to a big blender. Merge on high till smooth and then serve.

Nutrition: Calories: 99; Fat: 4 gm; Protein: 1 gm; Sodium: 1,348 mg; Fiber: 4 gm; Carbs: 16 gm; Sugar: 7 gm

105. Turkey Sweet Potato Hash

Preparation Time: ten mins

Cooking Time: twelve mins

Servings: four

Ingredients:

- 1 ½ tablespoon avocado oil
- one medium yellow onion, skinned and cubed
- 2 garlic pieces, crushed
- one medium sweet potato, cut into cubes (peeling not necessary)
- 1/2 pound lean ground turkey
- half tsp salt
- one tsp Italian seasoning blend

Directions:

1. Attach the oil and allow it to heat for one min. Include the onion and cook till softened, about five mins. Attach the garlic and cook for an additional thirty secs.
2. Include the sweet potato, turkey, salt, and Italian seasoning and cook for an extra five mins.

Nutrition: Calories: 172; Fat: 9 gm; Protein: 12 gm; Sodium: 348 mg; Fiber: 1 gm; Carbs: 10 gm; Sugar: 3 gm

106. Chicken Tenders with Honey Mustard Sauce

Preparation Time: five mins

Cooking Time: ten mins

Servings: four

Ingredients:

- one lb. chicken tenders
- one tbsp fresh thyme leaves
- half tsp salt
- quarter tsp black pepper
- one tbsp avocado oil
- one teacup chicken stock
- quarter teacup Dijon mustard
- quarter teacup raw honey

Directions:

1. Dry the chicken tenders with a towel and then season them with thyme, salt, and pepper.
2. Attach the oil and let it heat for two mins. Include the chicken tenders and seer them till brown on both sides, about one min on all sides. Press the Cancel button.
3. Take out the chicken tenders and set them aside. Include the stock to the pot. Use a spoon to scrape up any small bits from the bottom of the pot.
4. Set the steam rack in the inner pot and place the chicken tenders directly on the rack.
5. While the chicken is cooking, prepare the sauce.
6. In a container, blend the Dijon mustard and honey, then stir to blend.
7. Serve the chicken tenders with the honey mustard sauce.

Nutrition: Calories: 223; Fat: 5 gm; Protein: 22 gm; Sodium: 778 mg; Fiber: 0 gm; Carbs: 19 gm; Sugar: 18 gm

107. Chicken Breasts with Cabbage and Mushrooms

Preparation Time: ten mins

Cooking Time: eighteen mins

Servings: four

Ingredients:

- two tbsps avocado oil
- one lb. sliced Baby Bella mushrooms
- one and half tsps salt, divided
- 2 garlic pieces, crushed
- eight teacups severed green cabbage
- one and half tsps dried thyme
- half teacup chicken stock
- one and half lbs. boneless, skinless chicken breasts

Directions:

1. Include the oil. Allow it to heat for one min. Attach the mushrooms and quarter tsp of salt. Sauté till they have cooked down and released their liquid, about ten mins.
2. Include the garlic and sauté for an extra thirty secs. Press the Cancel button.
3. Attach the cabbage, quarter tsp of salt, thyme, and the stock to the inner pot. Stir to blend.
4. Dry the chicken breasts and sprinkle both sides with the rest of the salt. Place on top of the cabbage mixture.
5. Transfer to plates and spoon the juices on top.

Nutrition: Calories: 337; Fat: 10 gm; Protein: 44 gm; Sodium: 1,023 mg; Fiber: 4 gm; Carbs: 14 gm; Sugar: 2 gm

108. Duck with Bok Choy

Preparation Time: fifteen mins

Cooking Time: twelve mins

Servings: six

Ingredients:

- two tbsps coconut oil
- 1 onion, sliced thinly
- two tsps fresh ginger, grated finely
- 2 crushed garlic pieces
- one tbsp fresh orange zest, grated finely
- quarter teacup chicken broth
- two-third teacup fresh orange juice
- 1 roasted duck, meat picked
- 3 pounds bok choy leaves
- 1 orange, skinned, seeded, and segmented

Directions:

1. In a sizable griddle, melt the coconut oil on medium heat. Attach the onion, saute for around three mins. Include ginger and garlic then saute for around one-two mins.
2. Stir in the orange zest, broth, and orange juice.
3. Include the duck meat and cook for around three mins.
4. Transfer the meat pieces to a plate. Include the bok choy and cook for around three to four mins.
5. Divide the bok choy mixture into serving plates and top with duck meat.
6. Serve with the garnishing of orange segments.

Nutrition: Calories: 290; Fat: 4 gm; Fiber: 6 gm; Carbs: 8 gm; Protein: 14 gm

109. Beef with Mushroom and Broccoli

Preparation Time: sixty mins

Cooking Time: twelve mins

Servings: four

Ingredients:

For beef Marinade:

- 1 garlic piece, crushed
- 1 piece fresh ginger, crushed

- Salt and freshly ground black pepper
- three tbsps white wine vinegar
- three-quarter teacup beef broth
- one lb. flank steak, trimmed and sliced into thin strips

For vegetables:
- two tbsps coconut oil
- 2 garlic pieces
- three teacups broccoli rabe
- 4 oz. Shiitake mushrooms
- 8 oz. Cremini mushrooms

Directions:

For the marinade:
1. In a substantial container, mix all components except the beef. Include it and coat with the marinade generously. Refrigerate to soak for around 1/4 hour.
2. In a substantial griddle, warm oil on medium-high heat.
3. Detach the beef from the container, reserving the marinade.

For the vegetables:
1. Attach the beef and garlic and cook for around three to four mins or till browned.
2. In the same griddle, include the reserved marinade, broccoli, and mushrooms. Cook for approximately three to four mins.
3. Set in the beef and cook for around three to four mins.

Nutrition: Calories: 200; Carbs: 31 gm; Cholesterol: 93 mg; Fat: 4 gm; Protein: 10 gm; Fiber: 2 gm

110. **Beef with Zucchini Noodles**

Preparation Time: fifteen mins

Cooking Time: nine mins

Servings: four

Ingredients:
- one tsp fresh ginger, grated
- two medium garlic pieces, crushed
- quarter teacup coconut aminos
- two tbsps fresh lime juice
- one and half lbs. NY strip steak, trimmed and sliced thinly
- two medium zucchini, spiralized with blade C
- Salt as required
- three tbsps essential olive oil
- two medium scallions, sliced
- one tsp red pepper flakes, crushed
- two tbsps fresh cilantro, severed

Directions:
1. In a big container, merge ginger, garlic, coconut aminos, and lime juice. Include the beef and coat with

the marinade generously. Refrigerate to soak for approximately ten mins.
2. Set zucchini noodles over a big paper towel and sprinkle with salt.
3. Keep aside for around ten mins.
4. In a big griddle, heat oil on medium-high heat. Attach the scallions and red pepper flakes then sauté for around one min.
5. Attach the beef with the marinade and stir fry for around three to four mins or till browned.
6. Stir in the fresh cilantro, then include the zucchini and cook for approximately three to four mins.
7. Serve warm.

Nutrition: Calories: 1366; Carbs: 166 gm; Cholesterol: 6 mg; Fat: 67 gm; Protein: 59 gm; Fiber. 41 gm

111. **Spiced Ground Beef**

Preparation Time: ten mins

Cooking Time: twenty-two mins

Servings: five

Ingredients:
- two tbsps coconut oil
- 2 whole pieces
- 2 whole cardamoms
- 1 (2 inches) piece cinnamon stick
- two bay leaves
- one tsp cumin seeds
- 2 onions, severed
- Salt, as required
- half tbsp garlic paste
- half tbsp fresh ginger paste
- one lb. lean ground beef
- one and half tsps fennel seeds powder
- one tsp ground cumin
- one and half tsps red chili powder
- one-eighth tsp ground turmeric
- Freshly ground black pepper, as required
- one teacup coconut milk
- quarter teacup water
- quarter teacup fresh cilantro, severed

Directions:
1. In a sizable pan, warm oil on medium heat. Mix pieces, cardamoms, cinnamon, bay leaves, and cumin seeds: cook for around 20 seconds.
2. Attach the onion and 2 tweaks of salt then saute for around three to four mins.
3. Include the garlic-ginger paste and stir fry for around two mins.

4. Attach the beef and cook for around four-five mins, entering pieces using the spoon. Stir in spices and cook.

5. Set in the coconut milk and water: cook for around seven-eight mins. Flavor with salt and take away from the heat.

6. Serve hot using the garnishing of cilantro.

Nutrition: Calories: 216; Protein: 8.83 gm; Fat: 11.48 gm; Carbs: 21.86 gm

112. Ground Beef with Veggies

Preparation Time: sixty mins

Cooking Time: twenty-two mins

Servings: four

Ingredients:

- one-two tbsps coconut oil
- 1 red onion,
- 2 red Jalapeño peppers
- 2 crushed garlic pieces
- one lb. lean ground beef
- 1 small head broccoli, severed
- 1/2 head cauliflower
- 3 carrots, skinned and sliced
- 3 celery ribs
- Chopped fresh thyme, as required
- Dried sage, as required
- Ground turmeric, as required
- Salt and freshly ground black pepper

Directions:

1. Inside a big griddle, dissolve the coconut oil on medium heat.

2. Stir in the onion, jalapeño peppers, and garlic. Saute for around five mins.

3. Attach the beef and cook for around four-five mins, entering pieces using the spoon.

4. Include the rest of the components and cook, stirring occasionally for around eight-ten mins.

5. Serve warm.

Nutrition: Calories: 141; Cholesterol: 50 mg; Carbs: 6 gm; Fat: 1 gm; Sugar: 3 gm; Fiber: 2 gm

113. Ground Beef with Greens and Tomatoes

Preparation Time: fifteen mins

Cooking Time: fifteen mins

Servings: four

Ingredients:

- one tbsp organic olive oil
- 1/2 white onion, severed
- 2 garlic pieces, finely severed
- 1 Jalapeño pepper, finely severed
- one lb. lean ground beef
- one tsp ground coriander
- one tsp ground cumin
- half tsp ground turmeric
- half tsp ground ginger
- half tsp ground cinnamon
- half tsp ground fennel seeds
- Salt and freshly ground black pepper
- 8 fresh cherry tomatoes, quartered
- 8 collard green leaves, stemmed and severed
- one tsp fresh lemon juice

Directions:

1. In a big griddle, warm oil on medium heat.

2. Include the onion and saute for approximately 4 mins.

3. Stir in the garlic and jalapeño pepper. Saute for approximately one min.

4. Attach the beef and spices: cook for approximately six mins breaking into pieces while using a spoon.

5. Set in tomatoes and greens. Cook, stirring gently for around four mins.

6. Whisk in lemon juice and take away from the heat.

Nutrition: Calories: 444; Fat: 15 gm; Carbs: 20 gm; Fiber: 2 gm; Protein: 37 gm

Breakfast

114. Spinach Frittata

Preparation Time: ten mins

Cooking Time: thirty mins

Servings: four

Ingredients:

- two tsps olive oil
- one teacup red pepper, seeded and severed
- 1 garlic piece, crushed
- three teacups spinach leaves, severed
- four big eggs, beaten
- half tsp salt
- quarter teacup Parmesan cheese, freshly grated

Directions:

1. Warm up the oven to 350 **deg.F**. In a non-stick oven pan, heat one tsp of olive oil at middling temp.
2. Cook red peppers and garlic till vegetables are soft (about ten mins). In a medium container, blend the eggs, spinach, and salt: put away.
3. Include rest of the one tsp of olive oil into the pan with vegetables and include in the egg mixture.
4. Set the heat and cook for fifteen mins. Spray Parmesan cheese over the mixture and broil for an additional four mins.

Nutrition: Calories: 106; Fat: 8 gm; Carbs: 7 gm; Fiber: 2 gm; Protein: 3 gm

115. Banana and Pear Pita Pockets

Preparation Time: ten mins

Cooking Time: zero mins

Servings: one

Ingredients:

- 1/2 small banana, skinned and sliced
- 1 round Pita bread, made with refined white flour
- 1/2 small pear, skinned, seedless, cored, cooked, and sliced
- quarter teacup low-fat Cottage cheese

Directions:

1. Blend the banana, pear, and Cottage cheese in a small container. Slice the pita bread to make a pocket.
2. Fill it with the mixture.
3. Serve.

Nutrition: Calories: 402; Fat: 2 gm; Carbs: 87 gm; Fiber: 11 gm; Protein: 14 gm

116. Ripe Plantain Bran Muffins

Preparation Time: ten mins

Cooking Time: twenty mins

Servings: twelve

Ingredients:

- one and half teacups refined cereal
- two-third teacup low-fat milk
- four big eggs, lightly beaten
- quarter teacup canola oil
- two medium ripe plantains, mashed
- half teacup brown sugar
- one teacup refined white flour
- two tsps baking powder
- half tsp salt

Directions:

1. Warm up the oven to 400 **deg.F**. In a container, blend the bran cereal and milk; put away.
2. Include eggs and oil: stir in brown sugar and mashed ripe plantain. In another container, blend salt, flour, and baking powder.
3. Dissolve the dry components into the ripe plantain mixture, stir till blended.
4. Pour the batter evenly into paper-lined muffin tins: bake for eighteen mins or till golden brown and firm. Allow cooling prior to serving.

Nutrition: Calories: 325; Fat: 19 gm; Carbs: 37 gm; Fiber: 2 gm; Protein: 3 gm

117. Easy Breakfast Bran Muffins

Preparation Time: ten mins

Cooking Time: twenty mins

Servings: ten

Ingredients:

- two teacups refined cereal
- one teacup boiling water
- half teacup brown sugar
- half teacup butter
- 2 eggs
- 1/2-quart buttermilk
- two and half teacups refined white flour
- two and half tsps baking soda
- half tsp salt

Directions:

1. Warm up the oven to 400 deg.F. Soak one teacup of cereal in one teacup of boiling water and put away.
2. In a mixer, merge the brown sugar and butter till it is fully mixed. Include each egg separately and beat till fluffy. Then, stir in the buttermilk and the soaked cereal mixture.
3. In another container, blend salt, flour, and baking soda. Include the flour mixture into the batter and ensure not to over mix.
4. Include in the rest of the cup of cereal. Set the batter evenly into 10 greased or paper-lined muffin tins.

Bake for fifteen-twenty mins. Allow cooling prior to serving.

Nutrition: Calories: 440; Fat: 20 gm; Carbs: 57 gm; Fiber: 3 gm; Protein: 9 gm

118. Apple Oatmeal

Preparation Time: ten mins

Cooking Time: one-two mins

Servings: one

Ingredients:

- half teacup instant oatmeal
- three-quarter teacup milk or water
- half teacup apples, skinned and cooked pureed
- one tsp brown sugar

Directions:

1. In a microwave-safe container, mix oats, milk or water, and apples. Cook in a microwave on high.
2. Stir and cook for an extra thirty secs. Spray with brown sugar and include a splash of milk.

Nutrition: Calories: 295; Fat: 7 gm; Carbs: 47 gm; Fiber: 5 gm; Protein: 13 gm

119. Breakfast Burrito Wrap

Preparation Time: fifteen mins

Cooking Time: fifteen mins

Servings: one

Ingredients:

- one tbsp extra-virgin olive oil
- 2 slices turkey bacon
- quarter teacup green bell peppers, seeded and severed
- 2 eggs, beaten
- two tbsps milk
- quarter tsp salt
- two tbsps low-fat Monterrey Jack cheese, grated
- 1 white tortilla

Directions:

1. In a small non-stick pan, warm olive oil on medium heat and cook the turkey for around two mins till slightly crispy.
2. Attach bell peppers and continue to cook till warmed through. In a small container beat the eggs with milk and salt.
3. Gently, stir in your eggs till almost thoroughly cooked. Turn the heat down then include the cheese.
4. Cover and continue cooking till cheese has entirely melted. Place the mixture on the tortilla; then, roll it into a burrito.

Nutrition: Calories: 355; Fat: 2 gm; Carbs: 14 gm; Fiber: 4 gm; Protein: 23 gm

120. Zucchini Omelet

Preparation Time: fifteen mins

Cooking Time: fifteen mins

Servings: four

Ingredients:

- two tbsps extra-virgin olive oil
- one medium zucchini, seeded and cubed
- half medium tomato, seeded and severed
- four big eggs
- quarter teacup milk
- one tsp salt
- 4 whole-wheat English muffins

Directions:

1. Inside a big non-stick pan, warm olive oil over moderate heat. Include the zucchini and tomato.
2. Cook vegetables for five-ten mins or till they are soft.
3. In a separate container, merge the eggs, milk, and salt.
4. Attach the egg mixture to the pan and stir to cook through. Set with white English muffins.

Nutrition: Calories: 160; Fat: 10 gm; Carbs: 14 gm; Fiber: 2 gm; Protein: 6 gm

121. Coconut Chia Seed Pudding

Preparation Time: fifteen mins

Cooking Time: zero mins

Servings: two

Ingredients:

- 6 tablespoons Chia seeds
- two teacups coconut milk, unsweetened
- Blueberries for topping

Directions:

1. Mix well the chia seeds and milk. Refrigerate overnight.
2. Stir in the berries and serve.

Nutrition: Calories: 223; Fat: 12 gm; Carbs: 18 gm; Fiber: 2 gm; Protein: 10 gm

122. Spiced Oatmeal

Preparation Time: two mins

Cooking Time: two mins

Servings: two

Ingredients:

- one-third teacup quick oats
- quarter tsp ground ginger
- one-eighth tsp ground cinnamon
- A dash ground nutmeg
- A dash ground piece
- one tbsp almond butter
- one teacup water

Directions:

1. Blend the oats and water. Microwave for 45 seconds, then stir and cook for an extra 30-45 seconds.

2. Include in the spices and drizzle on the almond butter prior to serving.

Nutrition: Calories: 467; Fat: 11 gm; Carbs: 33 gm; Fiber: 4 gm; Protein: 6 gm

123. Breakfast Cereal

Preparation Time: five mins

Cooking Time: five mins

Servings: four

Ingredients:

- three teacups cooked old fashioned oatmeal
- three teacups cooked quinoa
- four teacups bananas, skinned and severed

Directions:

1. Blend the oatmeal and quinoa. Mix well.
2. Evenly, divide into 4 bowls and top with the bananas prior to serving.

Nutrition: Calories: 228; Fat: 3 gm; Carbs: 43 gm; Fiber: 6 gm; Protein: 12 gm

124. Sweet Potato Hash with Sausage and Spinach

Preparation Time: five mins

Cooking Time: fifteen mins

Servings: four

Ingredients:

- 4 small severed sweet potatoes
- 2 apples, cored and severed
- 1 garlic piece, crushed
- 1 pound ground sausage
- 10 oz. severed spinach
- Salt and pepper

Directions:

1. Brown the sausage till no pink remains. Include the rest of the components.
2. Cook till the spinach and apples are tender. Season as required. Serve warm.

Nutrition: Calories: 544; Fat: 2 gm; Carbs: 65 gm; Fiber: 2 gm; Protein: 11 gm

125. Cajun Omelet

Preparation Time: five mins

Cooking Time: eight mins

Servings: two

Ingredients:

- ¼ pound spicy sausage
- one-third teacup sliced mushrooms
- 1/2 cubed onion
- four big eggs
- half medium bell pepper, severed
- two tbsps water
- A tweak cayenne pepper (optional)

- Sea salt and fresh pepper as required
- one tbsp mustard

Directions:

1. Brown the sausage in a saucepan till thoroughly cooked. Include the mushrooms, onion, and bell pepper. Cook for an extra three-five mins, or till tender.
2. Meanwhile, whisk together the eggs, water, mustard, and spices. Season with salt and pepper.
3. Top with your eggs over then reduce to low heat. Cook till the top is nearly set and then fold the omelet in half and cover.
4. Cook for an extra minute prior to serving hot.

Nutrition: Calories: 467; Fat: 14 gm; Carbs: 11 gm; Fiber: 2 gm

126. Strawberry Cashew Chia Pudding

Preparation Time: ten mins

Cooking Time: zero mins

Servings: two

Ingredients:

- 6 tablespoons chia seeds
- two teacups cashew milk, unsweetened
- Strawberries, for topping

Directions:

1. Mix well the chia seeds and milk. Refrigerate overnight.
2. Stir in the berries and serve.

Nutrition:

Calories: 223; Fat: 12 gm; Carbs: 18 gm; Fiber: 2 gm; Protein: 10 gm

127. Peanut Butter Banana Oatmeal

Preparation Time: five mins

Cooking Time: zero mins

Servings: one

Ingredients:

- one-third teacup quick oats
- quarter tsp cinnamon (optional)
- 1/2 sliced banana
- one tbsp peanut butter, unsweetened

Directions:

1. Mix all components inside a container with a lid. Refrigerate.

Nutrition: Calories: 645; Fat: 32 gm; Carbs: 65 gm; Fiber: 5 gm; Protein: 26 gm

128. Overnight Peach Oatmeal

Preparation Time: ten mins

Cooking Time: zero mins

Servings: two

Ingredients:

- half teacup old fashioned oats
- two-third teacup skim milk

- half teacup plain Greek yogurt
- one tbsp chia seeds
- half tsp vanilla
- half teacup peach, skinned and cubed
- one medium banana, skinned and severed

Directions:
1. Blend the oats, milk, yogurt, chia seeds, and vanilla inside a container with a lid.
2. Refrigerate for twelve hrs.
3. Top with the fruits prior to serving.

Nutrition: Calories: 282; Fat: 6 gm; Carbs: 48 gm; Fiber: 2 gm; Protein: 10 gm

129. Mediterranean Salmon and Potato Salad

Preparation Time: fifteen mins

Cooking Time: eighteen mins

Servings: four

Ingredients:
- one lb. red potatoes, skinned and cut into wedges
- half teacup + two tbsps more extra-virgin olive oil
- two tbsps balsamic vinegar
- one tbsp fresh rosemary, crushed
- two teacups peas, cooked and drained
- 4 (4 oz. each) salmon fillets
- two tbsps lemon juice
- quarter tsp salt
- two teacups English cucumber, sliced and seedless

Directions:
1. Inside a saucepot, set water to a boil and cook potatoes till tender, about ten mins.
2. Drain and set potatoes back into the pan. To make the dressing, inside a container, set together half teacup of olive oil, vinegar, and rosemary.
3. Blend potatoes and peas with the dressing. Set aside. In a separate medium pan, warm the rest of the two tbsps of olive oil at middling temp.
4. Attach salmon fillets and set with lemon juice and salt.
5. Cook on both sides or till fish flakes easily. To serve, place cucumber slices on a serving plate top with potato salad and fish fillets.

Nutrition: Calories: 463; Fat: 4 gm; Carbs: 75 gm; Fiber: 18 gm; Protein: 34 gm

130. Celery Soup

Preparation Time: eight mins

Cooking Time: ten mins

Servings: two

Ingredients:
- one tbsp olive oil
- 3 garlic pieces, crushed
- two lbs. fresh celery, severed into one inch pieces
- six teacups vegetable stock
- one tsp salt

Directions:
1. Reserve celery tops for later use. Warmth up the oil at middling temp. in a soup pot.
2. Cook the garlic till softened, about three-five mins. Include celery stalks, salt, and vegetable stock then bring to a boil.
3. Cover and reduce the heat to low and simmer till the celery softens. Let the soup cool for a bit then puree with a hand blender.
4. Include and cook the celery tops on medium heat for five mins.

Nutrition: Calories: 51; Fat: 3 gm; Carbs: 4 gm; Fiber: 2 gm; Protein: 2 gm

131. Pea Tuna Salad

Preparation Time: fifteen mins

Cooking Time: zero mins

Servings: four

Ingredients:
- 3 pounds cooked peas
- half teacup low-fat mayonnaise
- one-third teacup tarragon vinegar
- one tsp honey Dijon mustard
- 2 small shallots, thinly sliced
- 2 (6 oz.) tuna cans, drained
- 2 small tarragon sprigs, finely severed

Directions:
1. Inside a big container, merge mayonnaise, vinegar, and mustard. Include tuna fish, shallots, and peas: toss to coat with dressing.
2. Secure and put in the fridge for one hr prior to serving. Set with fresh tarragon and serve.

Nutrition: Calories: 246; Fat: 13 gm; Carbs: 11 gm; Fiber: 1 gm; Protein: 22 gm

132. Vegetable Soup

Preparation Time: fifteen mins

Cooking Time: one hr twenty mins

Servings: two

Ingredients:
- two tbsps extra-virgin olive oil
- 4 garlic pieces, finely severed
- two celery stalks, finely sliced
- 2 carrots, finely sliced
- six teacups water or chicken broth
- quarter tsp thyme
- quarter tsp rosemary
- 1 bay leaf

- 1 can (14 oz.) peas
- half tsp salt

Directions:

1. Warmth up the oil at middling temp. in a soup pot. Include garlic, celery, and carrots and continue to cook for five mins, stirring occasionally.
2. Include water or chicken broth, thyme, rosemary, and bay leaf. Cook till it comes to a boil.
3. Set the heat and simmer gently for around forty-five to sixty mins. Include peas and season with salt.
4. Let soup cool slightly, take out the bay leaf and puree with a hand blender, till creamy.
5. Serve in warmed soup bowls.

Nutrition: Calories: 242; Fat: 8 gm; Carbs: 34 gm; Fiber: 13 gm; Protein: 12 gm

133. Carrot and Turkey Soup

Preparation Time: fifteen mins

Cooking Time: forty mins

Servings: four

Ingredients:

- 1/2 pound lean ground turkey
- 1/2 bag frozen carrot
- quarter teacup green peas
- 1 can (32 ounces) chicken broth
- two medium tomatoes, seeded and roughly severed
- one tsp garlic powder
- one tsp paprika
- one tsp oregano
- 1 bay leaf

Directions:

1. Over medium heat, set the ground turkey in a soup pot. Include peas, frozen carrot, paprika, tomatoes, garlic powder, bay leaf, oregano, and broth.
2. Set the pot to a boil, lower heat, cover, and simmer for thirty mins.

Nutrition: Calories: 436; Fat: 12 gm; Carbs: 20 gm; Fiber: 6 gm; Protein: 59 gm

134. Creamy Pumpkin Soup

Preparation Time: fifteen mins

Cooking Time: one hr ten mins

Servings: four

Ingredients:

- 1 pumpkin, cut lengthwise, seeds taken out, and skinned
- 1 sweet potato, cut lengthwise and skinned
- two tbsps olive oil
- 4 garlic pieces, unskinned
- four teacups vegetable stock
- quarter teacup light cream

- Salt
- one tbsp severed Shallots

Directions:

1. Warm up the oven to 375 deg.F. Cut all the sides of the pumpkin, shallots, and sweet potato with oil.
2. Transfer your vegetables with the garlic to a roasting pan. Set to roast for around forty mins or till tender.
3. Let the vegetables cool for a time and scoop out the flesh of the sweet potato and pumpkin.
4. In a soup pot, place the flesh of roasted vegetables, shallots, and skinned garlic. Include the broth and set to a boil.
5. Set the heat, and let it simmer, covered for thirty mins, stirring occasionally. Let the soup cool.
6. Set the soup with a hand blender, till smooth. Include the cream.
7. Season as required and simmer till warmed through, about five mins. Serve in warm soup bowls.

Nutrition: Calories: 332; Fat: 18 gm; Carbs: 32 gm; Fiber: 9 gm; Protein: 12 gm

135. Chicken Pea Soup

Preparation Time: fifteen mins

Cooking Time: fifty-five mins

Servings: four

Ingredients:

- one lb. chicken breast, skinless, boneless, and cubed
- two tbsps olive oil
- 3 garlic pieces, crushed
- 3 carrots, grated
- 1 bay leaf
- one tsp salt
- one tsp poultry seasoning
- eight teacups chicken broth
- half teacup dried split peas, washed and drained
- one teacup green peas

Directions:

1. Warmth up the olive oil at middling temp. in a soup pot. Include the chicken and cook for five mins, till lightly browned.
2. Attach the garlic, bay leaf, carrots, salt, and seasoning. Cook till vegetables soften, stirring occasionally.
3. Pour the broth and split peas into the pot: bring to a boil. Set the heat, cover, and simmer on low heat for thirty to forty-five mins.
4. Stir in green peas to the soup and heat for five mins, stirring to blend all components.

Nutrition: Calories: 176; Fat: 5 gm; Carbs: 18 gm; Fiber: 6 gm; Protein: 15 gm

136. Coconut Pancakes

Preparation Time: ten mins

Cooking Time: ten mins

Servings: two

Ingredients:

- half teacup coconut milk, plus additional as needed
- half tbsp maple syrup
- quarter teacup coconut flour
- half tsp salt
- 2 eggs
- half tbsp coconut oil or almond butter, plus additional for greasing the pan
- half tsp vanilla extract
- half tsp baking soda

Directions:

1. Using an electric mixer, blend the coconut milk, maple syrup, eggs, coconut oil, and vanilla in a medium mixing cup.
2. Blend the baking soda, coconut flour, and salt in a shallow mixing container.
3. Set the dry components with the wet components inside a blending container and beat till smooth and lump-free.
4. If the batter is too dense, include more liquid to thin it down to a typical pancake batter consistency.
5. Using coconut oil, lightly grease a big griddle or pan. Warm up the oven to medium-high.
6. Cook till golden brown on the rim for an extra two mins.
7. Continue cooking the leftover batter while stacking the pancake on a tray.

Nutrition: Calories: 193; Fat: 11 gm; Carbs: 15 gm; Sugar: 6 gm; Fiber: 6 gm; Protein: 9 gm; Sodium: 737 mg

Lunch

137. **Barbecue Beef Stir-Fry**

Preparation Time: five mins

Cooking Time: twenty-five mins

Servings: four

Ingredients:

- quarter teacup barbecue sauce
- three tbsps low-sodium beef broth
- one lb. boneless, cut into strips beef sirloin steak
- 1 sliced onion
- 1 thinly sliced carrot
- one tbsp oil
- two teacups hot cooked long-grain white rice

Directions:

1. Blend the broth and BBQ sauce into the container.
2. Rub one tablespoon of meat and let stand for five mins.
3. Include vegetable, meat, and oil into the griddle and cook at medium-high flame for four mins.

4. Include rest of the BBQ sauce mixture and blend well. Let simmer over medium-low flame for two mins.
5. Serve and relish!

Nutrition: Calories: 310; Carbohydrates: 34 gm; Protein: 23 gm; Fat: 9 gm

138. **Chicken Saffron Rice Pilaf**

Preparation Time: fifteen mins

Cooking Time: thirty mins

Servings: six

Ingredients:

- A tweak saffron
- one tbsp Ghee or olive oil
- 1 carrot, skinned, severed
- 1 celery stalk, outside parts skinned, severed
- one and half teacups Basmati rice or jasmine rice
- three teacups chicken broth, low-sodium
- one and quarter teacups chicken breast, roasted, shredded
- 1 lemon
- Fresh severed parsley, to garnish

Directions:

1. Include saffron and water into the container and soak it.
2. Include ghee into the griddle and heat it. Then, include celery and carrots and sauté for three to four mins till softened. Include rice and sauté till toasted.
3. Include saffron and chicken broth to the griddle, bring to a boil, lower the heat, and cook for twenty-five to thirty mins.
4. Include shredded chicken to the rice and toss to blend.
5. Let sit for five mins.
6. When ready to serve, include lemon juice over the rice.
7. Garnish with severed parsley leaves.

Nutrition: Calories: 269; Carbohydrates: 41 gm; Fats: 5 gm; Proteins: 13 gm

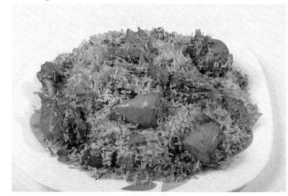

139. **Stir-Fry Ground Chicken and Green Beans**

Preparation Time: five mins

Cooking Time: five-ten mins

Servings: two

Ingredients:

- two teacups green beans
- one tbsp oil
- 1 slice ginger
- half lbs. ground chicken
- one tbsp soy sauce
- one tsp rice wine
- one tsp sesame oil
- one tsp sugar

Directions:

1. Include green beans into the boiled water. Cook till tender.
2. Drain it and put it into the container of ice water.
3. Include oil into the griddle and heat it. Then, include a ginger slice, and fry for one to two mins.
4. Include ground chicken. Cook till no longer pink.
5. Include sugar, sesame oil, rice wine, and soy sauce. Toss to blend.
6. Include drained green beans and cook them.
7. Serve and relish!

Nutrition: Calories: 162; Carbohydrates: 10 gm; Fats: 18 gm; Proteins: 22 gm; Fiber: 2 gm

140. Stewed Lamb

Preparation Time: five mins

Cooking Time: eight hrs

Servings: six

Ingredients:

- lamb leg, boneless
- two tbsps extra-virgin olive oil
- 400ml beef or vegetable broth
- 300 ml red wine
- 80 gm whole meal flour
- 400 gm button mushrooms, sliced in half
- one tsp fresh rosemary leaves
- 1kg potatoes, cut into quarters, red-skinned
- two celery sticks, severed
- 2 carrots, cut into big chunks
- one teacup parsley, severed

Directions:

1. Include olive oil into the saucepan and put it at medium flame.
2. Cook till browned. Include stock to the slow cooker, place the lamb with all components into the slow cooker, and cook on low flame for eight hours.
3. After eight hours, turn off the slow cooker and include cooled stock to the container to make a paste with whole meal flour. Stir well.

4. Include flour paste and sprinkle with pepper and salt.
5. Spray with fresh parsley leaves.

Nutrition: Calories: 481; Carbohydrates: 22 gm; Fats: 27 gm; Proteins: 28 gm; Fiber: 4 gm

141. Pulled Chicken Salad

Preparation Time: five mins

Cooking Time: five mins

Servings: four

Ingredients:

- 200 gm pulled BBQ chicken, cooked
- one-third teacup apricots, drained, thinly sliced
- 100 gm Orzo pasta
- 150 gm spinach, stalks taken out
- 70 gm Cheddar cheese, cut into small cubes
- 30 gm Parmesan cheese
- quarter teacup parsley, severed
- one-third teacup noodles
- 5 tablespoons olive oil
- three tbsps wine vinegar
- Salt and pepper, as required

Directions:

1. Shred cooked and cooled chicken with a fork.
2. Include cooked and cooled orzo pasta into the microwave dish. Top with parmesan cheese and microwave for one to two mins.
3. Include apricots, chicken, parsley, and spinach into the container and mix it well. Then, include red wine vinegar and olive oil, sprinkle with pepper and salt, and pour over the salad. Blend it well.
4. Include crispy noodles prior to serving.

Nutrition: Calories: 352; Carbohydrates: 14 gm; Fats: 19 gm; Proteins: 29 gm; Fiber: 3 gm

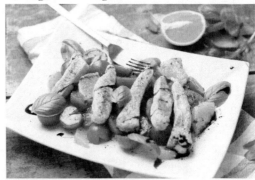

142. Lemongrass Beef

Preparation Time: five mins

Cooking Time: five-ten mins

Servings: four

Ingredients:

- two tbsps sesame oil

- one tbsp fish sauce
- two tbsps sweet chili sauce
- 2 packets Basmati rice, microwave
- two tsps coconut, shredded
- one tbsp lemongrass paste
- 500 gm beef, crushed, grass-fed
- one tbsp Thai seasoning
- 100 gm cucumber, skinned and cut into chunks
- 2 carrots, skinned and julienned
- quarter teacup basil, severed
- 1 lime, cut into four wedges

Directions:

1. Include sesame oil, lemongrass paste, fish sauce, and Thai seasoning into the wok and heat it. Include the crushed beef and stir well and cook for three to four mins till browned.
2. Cook the rice according to the instructions.
3. Include one teaspoon shredded coconut and stir well.
4. Include carrots, cucumber, rice, and crushed beef into the container.
5. Spray with Thai basil.
6. Pour sweet chili sauce and lime wedges over it.

Nutrition: Calories: 450; Carbohydrates: 50 gm; Fats: 19 gm; Proteins: 21 gm; Fiber: 3 gm

143. **Beetroot Carrot Salad**

Preparation Time: five mins
Cooking Time: forty mins
Servings: six
Ingredients:

- 3 beetroots, skinned
- 3 carrots, skinned
- 500 gm Halloumi, thickly sliced
- one tsp fresh oregano leaves
- 100 ml maple syrup
- 50 ml fresh lemon juice
- 50 gm spinach leaves
- 200 gm Tahini, hulled
- 100 gm noodles
- two tbsps extra virgin olive oil

Directions:

1. Warm up the oven to 180 deg.C.
2. Wrap the beetroot and carrots into the foil and put it into the oven for forty mins.
3. Let cool it, and then cut into the wedges.
4. Include olive oil into the saucepan and put it at medium flame.

5. Turn off the flame and include oregano, lemon juice, and maple syrup. Stir well.
6. Include one tablespoon of hulled tahini onto the plate.
7. Top with beetroot and carrot wedges, halloumi, and spinach leaves.
8. Spray with crispy noodles.

Nutrition: Calories: 206; Carbohydrates: 34.9 gm; Fats: 6.6 gm; Proteins: 4.5 gm; Fiber: 4 gm

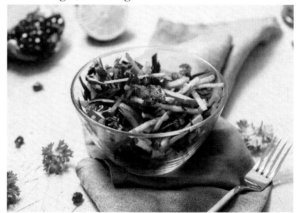

144. **Crunchy Maple Sweet Potatoes**

Preparation Time: five mins
Cooking Time: thirty mins
Servings: four
Ingredients:

- A tweak allspice
- two tbsps pure maple syrup
- quarter teacup cashew nuts, crushed

Potatoes:

- Extra-virgin olive oil spray
- 500 gm white potatoes, skinned
- 1 sweet potato, skinned
- quarter teacup plain white flour
- half teacup apple juice
- one tbsp butter
- one tsp sweet soy sauce
- one tbsp maple syrup
- A tweak cinnamon
- Salt and pepper, as required

Directions:

1. Warm up the oven to 180 deg.C.
2. Mix all components into the dish, place it into the oven, and bake for ten to fifteen mins till golden and crunchy.
3. Put it away.

Potatoes:

1. Let boil the potatoes for fifteen to twenty mins.
2. Spray the baking dish with extra virgin olive oil.

3. Slice potatoes into chunks and place them onto the dish.

4. Include all other components into the container. Blend them well.

5. Pour mixture over the potatoes and cover with a lid and bake for ten mins.

6. Spray with nuts.

Nutrition: Calories: 92; Carbohydrates: 18 gm; Fats: 2 gm; Proteins: 1.2 gm; Fiber: 1 gm

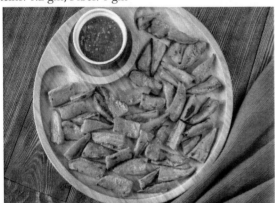

145. Veggie Bowl

Preparation Time: ten mins

Cooking time: ten mins

Servings: two

Ingredients:

- 100 gm white basmati rice
- 6 green beans
- Red pepper, skinned, cubed, and roasted
- ¼ ripe avocado, sliced lengthways
- half teacup cucumber, sliced
- 6 asparagus stems
- 1 tuna slice
- half teacup pumpkin chunks, skinned and roasted
- ½ lemon, cut into quarters
- two tsps ginger, pickled

Dressing:

- half teacup orange juice, freshly squeezed
- 4 tablespoons sesame oil
- A tweak salt and pepper

Directions:

1. Cook the rice and drain it well.
2. Blanche green beans.
3. Grill red pepper and take out the skin. Then, dice it.
4. Thinly slice the avocado lengthways.
5. Cut the cucumber thinly.
6. Drain six stems of asparagus.
7. Drain tuna slices of oil.
8. Boil the pumpkin chunks.

9. Place the red pepper in a mound in the middle of the plates.

10. Arrange all components on the plates.

11. Pour sesame oil over it. Spray with pepper and salt.

12. Pour dressing over the container.

Nutrition: Calories: 519; Carbohydrates: 59.2 gm; Fats: 28.4 gm; Proteins: 13.2 gm; Fiber: 5 gm

146. Pomegranate Salad

Preparation Time: five mins

Cooking Time: ten mins

Servings: four

Ingredients:

- one tsp chives, severed
- 300 gm zucchini
- 100 gm baby spinach
- 1 red pepper, skinned
- Extra-virgin olive oil spray

Dressing:

- three tbsps walnut oil
- quarter teacup pomegranate juice
- two tsps Dijon mustard
- Salt as required

Directions:

1. Include the entire components into the container and beat till blended for dressing.
2. Slice zucchini into chunks. Let chop the chives.
3. Spray the zucchini and chives with olive oil.
4. Place a frypan over medium flame.
5. Include chives and zucchini and fry till golden brown.
6. Then, include baby spinach leaves and stir well.
7. Turn off the flame. Pour dressing over the salad.

Nutrition: Calories: 273; Carbohydrates: 14.9 gm; Fats: 21.4 gm; Proteins: 9.5 gm; Fiber: 2 gm

147. Dijon Orange Summer Salad

Preparation Time: ten mins

Servings: two

Ingredients:

- 150 gm baby spinach leaves
- 2 oranges, skinned, deseeded, and sliced thinly
- 60 gm crushed macadamia nuts
- 100 gm feta cheese

Dressing:

- one tbsp thyme leaves
- 4 tablespoons extra-virgin olive oil
- one tbsp Dijon mustard
- 4 tablespoons lemon juice
- 2 crusty sourdough white bread rolls

Directions:

1. Include salad components into the container.
2. Include dressing components into the jar and shake it well.
3. Pour dressing over the salad. Blend it well.
4. Serve with a sourdough white bread roll.

Nutrition: Calories: 27; Carbohydrates: 6.7 gm; Proteins: 0.2 gm; Fiber: 3 gm

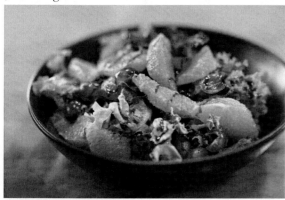

148. **Pulao Rice Prawns**

Preparation Time: five mins

Cooking Time: ten mins

Servings: four

Ingredients:

- 20 prawns, deveined, shelled
- three tbsps extra virgin olive oil
- 500ml water
- 200 ml coconut milk
- 3 cardamoms
- two bay leaves
- 1 tweak red chili powder
- half tsp turmeric powder
- quarter teacup fresh coriander, severed
- Black pepper as required
- 1 tweak garam masala powder
- 1 tweak asafoetida powder

Directions:

1. Include olive oil into the pan. Heat it. Then, include black pepper, cardamoms, bay leaves, and spices piece and cook for one to two mins till fragrant, about one to two mins.
2. Include cardamom, bay leaves, and pieces into the tea leaf ball.
3. Include asafetida powder, turmeric, garam masala, chili powder, salt, and prawns and blend well. Drain and include rice to the pan and cover with 500ml water and 200ml coconut milk.
4. Lower the heat and simmer till cooked thoroughly.
5. Garnish with fresh coriander leaves.

Nutrition: Calories: 424; Carbohydrates: 62 gm; Fats: 11 gm; Proteins: 19 gm; Fiber: 2 gm

149. **White Radish Crunch Salad**

Preparation Time: five mins

Servings: two

Ingredients:

- 200 gm radish, julienned
- 200 gm cucumber, shredded
- 50 gm noodles
- one tsp ginger, grated, steamed
- ¼ sheet nori, thinly sliced

Dressing:

- one tsp soy sauce
- one tsp rice vinegar
- one tsp maple syrup
- one tbsp orange juice
- one tbsp sesame oil

Directions:

1. Blend cucumber, ginger, and radish into the container. Pour dressing components over it. Top with nori and noodles. Stir well.
2. Serve!

Nutrition: Calories: 82; Carbohydrates: 5 gm; Fats: 7 gm; Proteins: 1 gm; Fiber: 2 gm

150. **Apple and Mushroom Soup**

Preparation Time: five mins

Cooking Time: five mins

Servings: two

Ingredients:

- 400 ml water
- ½ green apple, skinned, cored, and grated
- 100 gm pre-cooked rice noodles
- quarter teacup green chives, severed
- 2 mushrooms, sliced
- 100 gm silken tofu, crumbled
- 1 slice roasted seaweed

Directions:

1. Rinse the rice noodles in hot water and then strain them.
2. Include all components and stir for one to two mins.
3. Then, include crushed seaweed flakes.
4. Serve!

Nutrition:

Calories: 366; Carbohydrates: 41.1 gm; Fats: 19 gm; Proteins: 11 gm; Fibers: 3 gm

151. **Spring Watercress Soup**

Preparation Time: five mins

Cooking Time: twenty to twenty-five mins

Servings: four

Ingredients:

- 1 bunch watercress, rinsed
- one tbsp olive oil
- 1 green onion, cubed, green part only
- four teacups chicken stock
- four teacups baby arugula
- Sea salt as required
- one tbsp chives, snipped
- two tbsps greek yogurt

Directions:

1. Separate the dense and tough stems from the watercress leaves.
2. Dice the stems. Reserve the leaves.
3. Include oil to the pot or Dutch oven and put it at medium-high flame.
4. Then, include the green onion (green part only) and cubed watercress stems into the pot, lower the heat to medium, and sprinkle with salt.
5. Cook for five mins.
6. Include stock and bring to a boil over medium-high flame.
7. When boiled, lower the heat to medium-low and simmer for fifteen mins.
8. Include reserved watercress leaves and arugula and cook till wilted.
9. Turn off the flame.
10. Include soup into the immersion blender and blend till smooth.
11. Place soup back in the pan/pot and warm through.
12. Garnish with severed chives.

Nutrition: Calories: 174; Carbohydrates: 19 gm; Fats: 7 gm; Proteins: 10 gm

152. Oyster Sauce Tofu

Preparation Time: ten mins

Cooking Time: fifteen mins

Servings: four

Ingredients:

- 700 gm Tofu
- two tsps oil
- 1 slice ginger, skinned, crushed
- 1 scallion, trimmed, severed
- one and half teacups chicken broth or vegetable broth, low sodium
- three tbsps oyster sauce
- two tsps rice wine
- two tsps cornstarch
- one tsp water
- one tsp sesame oil

Directions:

1. Slice tofu into bite-sized squares. Put it away.
2. Include oil into the griddle and heat it.
3. Then, include ginger and green part of severed scallions. Cook for one to two mins.
4. Include tofu, rice wine, broth, and oyster sauce. Bring to a boil.
5. Lower the heat and to medium-low. Simmer for five mins.
6. Include water and cornstarch into the container. Stir to make a slurry.
7. Include tofu into the gravy and drizzle with sesame oil, and sprinkle with green parts of scallions.

Nutrition: Calories: 58; Carbohydrates: 4 gm; Fats: 3 gm; Proteins: 2 gm

153. Potato and Rosemary Risotto

Preparation Time: ten mins

Cooking Time: thirty mins

Servings: three

Ingredients:

- two tbsps olive oil
- 1 sprig rosemary, severed
- 1 green onion, cubed, green part only
- two-third teacup arborio rice
- 1 Yukon gold potato, rinsed, skinned scrubbed, and cubed
- three and half teacups chicken stock, low-sodium
- one tbsp Parmesan cheese, grated
- one tsp butter
- Salt and pepper, as required

Directions:

1. Include olive oil into the Dutch oven and heat it over medium-high flame.
2. Include rosemary and cook for one min. Then, include green onion and cook for two mins till translucent.
3. Turn the heat down to medium and sprinkle with salt. Let sweat for eight mins.
4. Take out the lid and elevate the heat to medium-high and then include rice to it. Blend it well.
5. Include potato and cook for one min more.
6. Include chicken stock and bring to a boil.
7. Lower the heat to low and simmer for twenty mins till al dente.
8. Include butter and parmesan cheese and turn off the flame.
9. Let sit for five mins.
10. Include more stock if needed.
11. Spray with black pepper.

Nutrition: Calories: 377; Carbohydrates: 55 gm; Fats: 13 gm; Proteins: 12 gm

154. Cheesy Baked Tortillas

Preparation Time: ten mins

Cooking Time: forty mins

Servings: four

Ingredients:

- 255 gm pizza sauce
- 20 ml extra-virgin olive oil
- Extra-virgin olive oil spray
- Plain Greek yogurt, as needed
- 1 lime juice
- one tsp onion powder
- half tsp sweet paprika
- 250 gm cheddar cheese, low-fat
- 250 gm chicken, cooked, shredded
- 400 gm white potato, skinned
- 400 gm basmati rice, cooked and drained
- Salt and pepper, as required
- 6 flour tortillas

Directions:

1. Warm up the oven to 210 deg.C.
2. Spray the potatoes with olive oil spray.
3. Spray with paprika powder and place it into the oven and bake for twenty mins.
4. Include onion powder and olive oil into the pan and heat it for one min.
5. Include tofu or chicken, 180 gm of pizza sauce, pepper, salt, and lemon juice, and blend well.
6. Layout tortillas onto the clean surface and top with chicken or tofu mixture, rice, and baked potatoes and top with cheese.
7. Roll the burritos and place them onto the dish.
8. Top with rest of the cheese and bake for fifteen to twenty mins.

Nutrition: Calories: 389; Carbohydrates: 31 gm; Fats: 20 gm; Proteins: 22 gm; Fiber: 4 gm

155. Smoky Rice

Preparation Time: ten mins

Cooking Time: twenty mins

Servings: four

Ingredients:

- 400 gm white basmati rice
- 200 ml pasta
- ½ green onion, skinned and severed, green part only
- ¼ red capsicum, severed
- 4 tablespoons extra-virgin olive oil
- 70 gm tomato puree
- 3 bay leaves
- one tsp paprika
- one tsp cumin
- A tweak black pepper
- A tweak chili
- 4 tablespoons coconut oil
- Banana, skinned and severed
- Salt, as required

Directions:

Rice:

1. Rinse rice and soak for twenty mins.
2. Let boil it for five mins. Then, drain it.
3. Include black pepper, paprika, cumin, chili, half green onion (green part only), pasta, and red capsicum into the blender and blend till smooth.
4. Include oil into the saucepan and put it at medium flame.
5. Include capsicum mixture to the pan and sprinkle with salt; cook for a couple of mins till fragrant. Then, include tomato puree and bay leaves, and cook for five mins.
6. Include drained rice and one cup of water and simmer for eight mins till the rice is soft. Discard bay leaves. Put it away.

Banana:

1. Include coconut oil and banana into the pan. Cook till golden.
2. Include banana over the rice.
3. Serve!

Nutrition: Calories: 447; Carbohydrates: 69 gm; Fats: 11 gm; Proteins: 11 gm; Fiber: 3 gm

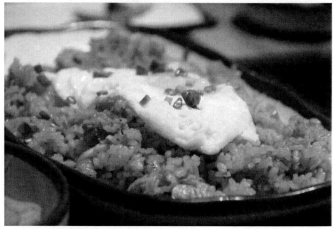

156. Zucchini Lasagna

Preparation Time: ten mins

Cooking Time: forty mins

Servings: four

Ingredients:

- 800 gm zucchini, grated
- one tsp green onion, green part only
- one tbsp chives, severed

- one tbsp dried oregano
- 250 gm Ricotta, low-fat
- 50 gm Cheddar cheese, low-fat, and shredded
- 350 ml Passata
- 9 dried Lasagna sheets, gluten-free
- Extra virgin oil, as needed
- Salt and pepper, as required

Instructions:

1. Warm up the oven to 210 deg.C.
2. Include olive oil into the frying pan and heat it.
3. Include green onion and zucchini and cook for three mins.
4. Lower the heat, include 25 gm of low-fat cheddar cheese and ricotta, and sprinkle with pepper and salt. Put it away.
5. Let boil the lasagna sheet in the salted water for five to six mins.
6. Then, drain it. Include some olive oil to the pasta.
7. Place lasagna sheet onto the baking dish, include ricotta and zucchini mixture, and sprinkle with fresh chives and oregano. Then, include tomato passata.
8. Lower the heat of the oven to 180 deg.C.
9. Bake the lasagna for thirty mins.
10. Serve with salad.

Nutrition: Calories: 362; Carbohydrates: 7 gm; Fats: 26 gm; Proteins: 25 gm; Fiber: 3 gm

157. **Greek Chicken Skewers**

Preparation Time: twenty mins

Cooking Time: twenty mins

Additional time: two hrs

Servings: four

Ingredients:

- quarter teacup lemon juice
- quarter teacup wok oil
- 1/8 cup red wine vinegar
- one tbsp onion flakes
- one tbsp garlic, crushed
- 1 lemon, zested
- one tsp Greek seasoning
- one tsp poultry seasoning
- one tsp dried oregano
- one tsp ground black pepper
- half tsp dried thyme
- 3 chicken breasts, cut into one inch pieces, skinless and boneless

Directions:

1. Whisk the thyme, pepper, oregano, poultry seasoning, Greek seasoning, lemon zest, garlic, onion flakes, vinegar, oil, and lemon juice into the container. Place them into the re-sealable plastic bag.
2. Include chicken and coat with marinade and seal the bag. Place it into the fridge for two hours.
3. Warm up the oven to 350 deg.F.
4. Discard marinade and thread chicken onto the skewers.
5. Place skewers onto the baking sheet.
6. Cook for twenty mins till golden brown.

Nutrition: Calories: 248; Carbohydrates: 4.1 gm; Protein: 18.1 gm; Fat: 17 gm

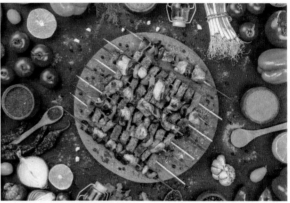

158. **Roast Beef**

Preparation Time: five mins

Cooking Time: one hr

Servings: six

Ingredients:

- 3 pounds beef eye round roast
- half tsp Kosher salt
- half tsp garlic powder
- quarter tsp freshly ground black pepper

Directions:

1. Warm up the oven to 375 deg.F.
2. Place roast into the pan and sprinkle with pepper, garlic powder, and salt. Cook it into the oven for one hour.
3. Let cool it for fifteen to twenty mins.
4. Serve and relish!

Nutrition: Calories: 48; Carbohydrates: 0.2 gm; Protein: 44.8 gm; Fat: 32.4 gm

159. **Banana Cake**

Preparation Time: twenty mins

Cooking Time: one hr fifteen mins

Servings: fifteen

Ingredients:

- one and one-third teacups bananas, mashed
- 2 ½ tablespoons lemon juice
- one and half teacups milk
- three teacups flour

- one and half tsps baking soda
- quarter tsp salt
- two-third teacup butter, softened
- one teacup white sugar
- half teacup brown sugar
- 3 eggs
- one tsp vanilla

Frosting:

- 8 oz. cream cheese
- one-third teacup butter, softened
- three and half teacups powdered sugar
- one tsp lemon juice
- one and half tsps lemon zest from 1 lemon

Directions:

1. Warm up the oven to 350 deg.F. Grease and flour the pan.
2. Include 1 ½ tablespoons lemon juice into the cup. Then, include one and a half cups milk, and keep it aside.
3. Blend one tablespoon lemon juice and mashed banana. Put it away.
4. Include white sugar, brown sugar, and butter into the container and beat it well.
5. Include eggs and vanilla and blend at high speed till fluffy.
6. Mix the salt, baking soda, and flour into the container.
7. Include flour mixture and milk to the egg mixture and stir well.
8. Then, fold it into the bananas. Place mixture into the pan.
9. Bake it for one hour and ten mins.
10. When done, place it into the freezer for forty-five mins.

To prepare the frosting:

1. Cream the cream cheese and butter into the container. Include lemon juice and lemon zest. Blend well.
2. Include powdered sugar and stir well. Top frosting over the cake.

Nutrition: Calories: 470; Carbohydrates: 70 gm; Protein: 5 gm; Fat: 19 gm

160. Grilled Fish Steaks

Preparation Time: ten mins

Cooking Time: ten mins

Additional time: one hr ten mins

Servings: two

Ingredients:

- 1 garlic piece, crushed
- 6 tablespoons olive oil
- one tsp dried basil

- one tsp salt
- one tsp ground black pepper
- one tbsp lemon juice
- one tbsp fresh parsley, severed
- 6 oz. Halibut fillets

Directions:

1. Mix the parsley, lemon juice, pepper, salt, basil, olive oil, and garlic into the container.
2. Include halibut fillets into the glass dish and place marinade over it.
3. Place it into the fridge for one hour.
4. Oil the grate and preheat the grill on high heat.
5. Discard marinade and place halibut fillets onto the grill, and cook for five mins on all sides.
6. When done, serve and relish!

Nutrition: Calories: 554; Carbohydrates: 2.2 gm; Protein: 36.3 gm; Fat: 43.7 gm

161. Apple Pudding

Preparation Time: ten mins

Cooking Time: thirty mins

Servings: six

Ingredients:

- half teacup butter, melted
- one teacup white sugar
- one teacup all-purpose flour
- two tsps baking powder
- quarter tsp salt
- one teacup milk
- two teacups apple, severed and skinned
- one tsp ground cinnamon

Directions:

1. Warm up the oven to 375 deg.F.
2. Mix the milk, salt, baking powder, flour, sugar, and butter into the baking dish.
3. Mix the cinnamon and apples into the container and microwave it for two to five mins. Place apple into the middle of the batter.
4. Place it into the oven and bake for a half-hour.
5. Serve and relish!

Nutrition: Calories: 384; Carbohydrates: 57.5 gm; Protein: 3.8 gm; Fat: 16 gm

162. Lamb Chops

Preparation Time: thirty mins

Cooking Time: thirty mins

Servings: two

Ingredients:

- 2lb Lamb chops, cut ¾" dense, 4 pieces
- Kosher salt and Black pepper for seasoning
- one tbsp garlic, crushed

- two tbsps rosemary, severed
- two tbsps thyme, severed
- half tsp parsley, severed
- quarter teacup extra-virgin olive oil

Directions:
1. Rub the lamb chops with pepper and salt.
2. Mix the two tablespoons olive oil, parsley, thyme, rosemary, and garlic into the container.
3. Rub this paste on each side of the lamb chops and let marinate it for a half-hour.
4. Place two tbsps of olive oil into the frying pan over medium-high flame.
5. Include lamb chops and cook for two to three mins.
6. Flip and cook for three to four mins more.
7. Let cool it for ten mins.
8. Serve and relish!

Nutrition: Calories: 465; Carbohydrates: 12 gm; Protein: 14 gm; Fat: 38 gm

163. Eggplant Croquettes

Preparation Time: fifteen mins
Cooking Time: twenty mins
Servings: six
Ingredients:
- 2 eggplants, skinned and cubed
- one teacup cheddar cheese, shredded
- one teacup Italian seasoned bread crumbs
- 2 eggs, beaten
- two tbsps dried parsley
- two tbsps onion, severed
- 1 piece garlic, crushed
- one teacup vegetable oil, for frying
- one tsp salt
- half tsp ground black pepper

Directions:
1. Microwave the eggplant over medium-high heat for three mins.
2. Flip and cook for two mins more.
3. If eggplant did not tender, cook for two mins more.
4. Then, drain it and mash the eggplants.
5. Mix the salt, garlic, onion, parsley, eggs, cheese, breadcrumbs, and mashed eggplant.
6. Make the patties from the eggplant mixture.
7. Include oil into the griddle and heat it. Place eggplant patties into the griddle and fry till golden brown for five mins.
8. Serve and relish!

Nutrition: Calories: 266; Carbohydrates: 23.6 gm; Protein: 12 gm; Fat: 14.4 gm

164. Cucumber Egg Salad

Preparation Time: ten mins
Cooking Time: fifteen mins
Servings: four
Ingredients:
- 4 eggs
- 4 cucumbers, seedless
- 4 dill pickles
- three tbsps mayonnaise

Directions:
1. Include eggs into the saucepan and cover it with cold water. Let boil it.
2. Take out from the flame. Let stand eggs in hot water for ten to twelve mins.
3. Take out from the hot water and cool it.
4. Peel eggs and chop them. Include it into the salad container.
5. Cube the cucumber and include to the eggs.
6. Include mayonnaise and blend it well.
7. Place it into the fridge till chill.

Nutrition: Calories: 176; Carbohydrates: 8 gm; Protein: 7.6 gm; Fat: 13.4 gm

Snacks

165. Papaya-Mango Smoothie

Preparation Time: five mins
Cooking Time: zero mins
Servings: two
Ingredients:
- one teacup mango, cubed
- one teacup papaya chunks
- one teacup almond or lactose-free milk
- one tbsp honey or maple syrup

Directions:
1. Blend all components in a blender. Then, pulse till smooth.
2. Pour into a big glass. Relish!

Nutrition: Calories: 554; Fat: 32 gm; Carbs: 14 gm; Sugar: 8 gm; Fiber: 2 gm; Protein: 50 gm; Sodium: 632 mg

166. Cantaloupe Smoothie

Preparation Time: five mins
Cooking Time: zero mins
Servings: two
Ingredients:
- one teacup cantaloupe, cubed
- half teacup vanilla yogurt or lactose-free yogurt
- half teacup of orange juice
- one tbsp honey or maple syrup
- 2 ice cubes

Directions:

1. Merge all components in a blender. Then, pulse till smooth.
2. Pour into a big glass.
3. Relish!

Nutrition: Calories: 179; Fat: 13 gm; Carbs: 6 gm; Sugar: 3 gm; Fiber: 1 gm; Protein: 10 gm; Sodium: 265 mg

167. Cantaloupe-Mix Smoothie

Preparation Time: five-ten mins

Cooking Time: zero mins

Servings: two

Ingredients:

- one teacup cantaloupe, cubed
- half teacup mango, cubed
- half teacup almond milk or lactose-free cow milk
- half teacup of orange juice
- two tbsps lemon
- one tbsp honey or maple syrup
- 2 ice cubes

Directions:

1. Mix all components in a blender till smooth.
2. Pour into a big glass.
3. Relish!

Nutrition: Calories: 329; Fat: 17 gm; Carbs: 9 gm; Sugar: 3 gm; Fiber: 5 gm; Protein: 37 gm; Sodium: 430 mg

168. Applesauce-Avocado Smoothie

Preparation Time: five-ten mins

Cooking Time: zero mins

Servings: one

Ingredients:

- one teacup unsweetened almond or lactose-free milk
- 1/2 avocado
- half teacup applesauce
- quarter tsp ground cinnamon
- half teacup ice
- half tsp stevia or one tbsp honey, for sweetness (optional)

Directions:

1. Blend all components in a blender. Pulse the mix till smooth.
2. Pour into a big glass.
3. Relish!

Nutrition: Calories: 270; Fat: 11 gm; Carbs: 4 gm; Sugar: 1 gm; Fiber: 1 gm; Protein: 39 gm; Sodium: 664 mg

169. Pina Colada Smoothie

Preparation Time: five-ten mins

Cooking Time: zero mins

Servings: one

Ingredients:

- one teacup papaya chunks
- half teacup unsweetened almond milk or lactose-free milk
- 1 banana
- half tsp vanilla extract, as required
- one tbsp honey, maple syrup, or one tsp stevia (optional)

Directions:

1. Blend all components in a blender and then pulse till smooth and creamy.
2. Pour into a big glass.
3. Relish!

Nutrition: Calories: 329; Fat: 17 gm; Carbs: 9 gm; Sugar: 3 gm; Fiber: 5 gm; Protein: 37 gm; Sodium: 430mg

170. Diced Fruits

Preparation Time: ten mins

Cooking Time: forty mins

Servings: six

Ingredients:

- 4 peaches, skin taken out and thinly sliced
- one lb. apple, pitted and skin taken out
- one tsp cinnamon powder
- one teacup honey or maple syrup
- one tsp vanilla extract

Directions:

1. Inside a big pot, cook the fruits in boiling water at middling temp. till softened.
2. Inside a big container, mix well all components (except the fruits).
3. Pour the syrup over fruits and let the compote be thickened.
4. Pour the compote into a jar. Serve hot or cold.
5. Relish!

Nutrition: Calories: 178; Fat: 4 gm; Carbs: 7 gm; Fiber: 2 gm; Protein: 27 gm

171. Applesauce

Preparation Time: ten mins

Cooking Time: thirty mins

Servings: four

Ingredients:

- 6 organic apples, skinned, cored, and cubed
- half teacup boiling water
- half tsp cinnamon powder
- quarter teacup sugar or 4 tablespoons honey
- two tbsps fresh lemon juice
- quarter tsp salt

Directions:

1. Inside a big pot, cook apples with boiling water, lemon juice, cinnamon, sugar, or honey, and salt over

medium-low heat till softened. Take out from the heat.

2. You can mash all components by using a fork or blend with a blender or a food processor.

3. Pour the applesauce into a suitable container or jar. Serve warm or cold.

4. Relish!

Nutrition: Calories: 51; Fat: 3 gm; Carbs: 4 gm; Fiber: 2 gm; Protein: 2 gm

172. Avocado Dip

Preparation Time: ten mins

Cooking Time: zero mins

Servings: four

Ingredients:

- 6 avocados, skinned
- half tbsp extra-virgin olive oil
- quarter teacup severed fresh cilantro
- two tbsps fresh lime juice
- one tsp fresh lemon juice
- half tsp salt

Directions:

1. Inside a big container, set avocados with a fork.

2. Include extra-virgin olive oil and the other components.

3. Relish!

Nutrition: Calories: 75; Carbs: 0.1 gm; Protein: 13.4 gm; Fat: 1.7 gm; Sugar: 0 gm; Sodium: 253 mg

173. Homemade Hummus

Preparation Time: ten mins

Cooking Time: sixty mins

Servings: four

Ingredients:

- 1/4 pound dried chickpeas (soaked in water for a night)
- one and half tbsps tahini
- one tbsp lemon juice
- two tbsps extra-virgin olive oil, divided
- quarter tsp cumin powder
- half tsp salt
- one tbsp water
- one tsp baking soda (optional)
- one tsp paprika powder (optional)

Directions:

1. First, you need to soak the chickpeas overnight in water and optionally include baking soda to the water.

2. Cook your chickpeas in a big pot with water, at middling temp. for around one hr. Check if they are cooked well by crushing one of them with a fork in your hand.

3. When chickpeas are cooked, drain and put them in a blender.

4. Include one tbsp of extra-virgin olive oil, lemon juice, tahini, cumin powder, and salt to the blender. Blend till your hummus gets a soft, creamy texture equally.

5. Spray with one tbsp of extra-virgin olive oil or paprika powder (optional).

6. Serve immediately or fridge it.

Nutrition: Calories: 207; Fat: 16 gm; Carbs: 5 gm; Sugar: 2 gm; Fiber: 1 gm; Protein: 12 gm; Sodium: 366 mg

174. Tofu

Preparation Time: ten mins

Cooking Time: twenty-five mins

Servings: four

Ingredients:

- one and half teacups firm tofu, pressed and drained
- 1 avocado, cubed
- one tbsp extra-virgin olive oil
- Salt and pepper, as required

Directions:

1. Warm up your oven to 400 deg.F.

2. Choose a baking sheet, cover it with parchment paper or spray extra-virgin olive oil. Cut tofu cubes of 1/2 inch and spray extra-virgin olive oil on them.

3. Let it bake for fifteen mins till golden brown and crispy. Flip tofu and cook for an extra ten mins. Take out from the oven. Let it rest for ten mins.

4. Cube the avocado on a plate. Include salt and pepper.

5. Mix the tofu with avocado inside a container. Relish!

Nutrition: Calories: 645; Fat: 32 gm; Carbs: 65 gm; Fiber: 5 gm; Protein: 26 gm

175. Almond Butter Sandwich

Preparation Time: ten mins

Cooking Time: five mins

Servings: one

Ingredients:

- 2 slices white bread or white gluten-free bread
- one tbsp organic smooth almond butter

Directions:

1. Set 1 piece of bread with almond butter.

2. Toast and relish!

Nutrition: Calories: 178; Fat: 4 gm; Carbs: 7 gm; Fiber: 2 gm; Protein: 27 gm

176. Gluten-Free Muffins

Preparation Time: fifteen mins

Cooking Time: thirty mins

Servings: ten-fifteen

Ingredients:

- two tbsps extra-virgin olive oil
- two and half teacups almond flour, blanched

- 3 big organic free-range eggs
- quarter teacup organic maple syrup
- two tsps vanilla extract
- quarter teacup banana, mashed
- one tsp lemon juice
- 3/4 teaspoon baking soda
- quarter tsp cinnamon powder
- half tsp salt

Directions:

1. Warm up your oven to 375 deg.F.
2. In a container, set almond flour, cinnamon, baking soda, and salt. Mix well.
3. In another container, include extra-virgin olive oil, vanilla extract, eggs, ripe banana, maple syrup, and lemon juice. Whisk well.
4. Mix both bowls and stir with a wooden spoon till the flour is mixed well with the other components.
5. Prepare 10 muffin cups. Pour them to the top and then bake for fifteen mins.
6. To avoid browning quickly, loosely cover muffins with aluminum foil. Cook for an extra fifteen mins.
7. Put a toothpick in a muffin to check if it cooks well or not. If cooked well, the toothpick should not stick to the muffin.
8. Take out from the oven. Let the muffins cool for additional fifteen mins. Relish!

Nutrition: Calories: 408; Fat: 26 gm; Carbs: 4 gm; Sugar: 1 gm; Fiber: 1 gm; Protein: 47 gm; Sodium: 426 mg

Dinner

177. Italian Style Stuffed Zucchini Boats

Preparation Time: ten mins

Cooking Time: twenty-five mins

Servings: two

Ingredients:

- 6 big zucchini
- half tbsp olive oil
- Kosher salt
- Freshly ground black pepper
- quarter tsp garlic powder
- 1 small yellow onion, cubed
- 2 garlic pieces, crushed
- one lb. ground turkey
- 1 (28 ounces) can crush tomatoes
- 4 ounces Mozzarella cheese, shredded
- 1 ounce Parmesan cheese, freshly grated
- Flat-leaf parsley for garnishing
- Cooking spray

Directions:

1. Turn your oven on and allow to preheat up to 425 deg.F and lightly grease a 9x13-inch baking dish with cooking spray.
2. Divide the zucchini in half lengthwise and then scoop out the seeds. Brush with olive oil and season with salt, pepper and garlic powder.
3. Roast in the prepared dish for twenty mins, or till it begins to soften.
4. Meanwhile, saute the onions and garlic in half tbsp of olive oil over medium-high heat in a big griddle.
5. Cook for three to four mins, then include the ground turkey and brown. Attach the tomatoes and bring them to a boil.
6. Reduce the heat to medium and then let simmer till the zucchini is done. Stir in half tsp salt and pepper as required.
7. Set to bake for around five mins or almost till the Mozzarella cheese you added has melted about three-five mins.
8. Serve hot, garnished with Parmesan cheese and parsley.

Nutrition: Calories: 2981; Fat: 7 gm; Carbs: 14 gm; Fiber: 2 gm; Protein: 25 gm

178. Chicken Cutlets

Preparation Time: ten mins

Cooking Time: fifteen mins

Servings: four

Ingredients:

- 4 teaspoons red wine vinegar
- two tsps crushed garlic pieces
- two tsps dried sage leaves
- one lb. chicken breast cutlets
- Salt and pepper, as required
- quarter teacup refined white flour
- two tsps olive oil

Directions:

1. Set a good amount of plastic wrap on the kitchen counter: sprinkle with half the blended sage, garlic and vinegar.
2. Put the chicken breast on the plastic wrap: sprinkle with the rest of the vinegar mixture. Season lightly with pepper and salt.
3. Secure the chicken with the second sheet of plastic wrap. Use a kitchen mallet to pound the breast till it is flattened. Let stand five mins.
4. Set the chicken on both sides with flour. In a griddle, heat the oil at middling temp.
5. Include half of the chicken breast and cook for 1 ½ minute or till it is browned on the bottom.
6. Turn on the other side and let it cook for three mins.
7. Take out the chicken breast and place it on an oven-proof serving plate so that you can keep warm.

8. Reduce the liquid by half. Pour the mixture over the chicken breast: serve immediately.

Nutrition: Calories: 549; Fat: 6 gm; Carbs: 7 gm; Fiber: 1 gm; Protein: 114 gm

179. Slow Cooker Salsa Turkey

Preparation Time: eight mins

Cooking Time: seven hrs

Servings: four

Ingredients:

- two lbs. turkey breasts, boneless and skinless
- one teacup salsa
- one teacup small tomatoes, cubed, canned choose low-sodium
- two tbsps taco seasoning
- half teacup celery, finely cubed
- half teacup carrots, shredded
- three tbsps low-fat sour cream

Directions:

1. Include the turkey to your slow cooker. Season it with taco seasoning then top with salsa and vegetables.
2. Include in half teacup of water. Set to cook on low for seven hrs (internal temp. should be 165 deg.F when done).
3. Shred the turkey with 2 forks, include in sour cream, and stir. Relish.

Nutrition: Calories: 178; Fat: 4 gm; Carbs: 7 gm; Fiber: 2 gm; Protein: 27 gm

180. Sriracha Lime Chicken and Apple Salad

Preparation Time: ten mins

Cooking Time: fifteen mins

Servings: four

Ingredients:

Sriracha Lime Chicken:

- 2 organic chicken breasts
- three tbsps sriracha
- 1 lime, juiced
- quarter tsp fine sea salt
- quarter tsp freshly ground pepper
- Fruit Salad:
- 4 apples, skinned, cored, and cubed
- one teacup organic grape tomatoes
- one-third teacup red onion, finely severed
- Lime Vinaigrette:
- one-third teacup light olive oil
- quarter teacup apple cider vinegar
- 2 limes, juiced
- A dash of fine sea salt

Directions:

1. Use salt and pepper to season the chicken on both sides. Spread on the sriracha and lime and let sit for twenty mins.
2. Cook the chicken on all sides at middling temp., or till done. Grill the apple with the chicken.
3. Meanwhile, whisk together the dressing and season as required.
4. Arrange the salad, topping it with red onion and tomatoes.
5. Serve as a side to the chicken and apple.

Nutrition: Calories: 484; Fat: 28 gm; Carbs: 32 gm; Fiber: 8 gm; Protein: 30 gm

181. Pan-Seared Scallops with Lemon-Ginger Vinaigrette

Preparation Time: ten mins

Cooking Time: ten mins

Servings: two

Ingredients:

- one lb. sea scallops
- one tbsp extra-virgin olive oil
- quarter tsp sea salt
- two tbsps lemon-ginger vinaigrette
- A tweak of freshly ground black pepper

Directions:

1. Heat the olive oil in a non-stick griddle or pan over medium-high heat till it starts shimmering.
2. Include the scallops to the griddle or pan after seasoning them with pepper and salt. Cook for three mins on all sides or till the fish is only opaque.
3. Serve with a dollop of vinaigrette on top.

Nutrition: Calories: 280; Fat: 16; Carbs: 5 gm; Sugar: 1 gm; Fiber: 0 gm; Protein: 29 gm; Sodium: 508 mg

182. Roasted Salmon and Asparagus

Preparation Time: five mins

Cooking Time: fifteen mins

Servings: two

Ingredients:

- one tbsp extra-virgin olive oil
- one lb. salmon, cut into 2 fillets
- 1/2 lemon zest and slices
- 1/2 pound asparagus spears, trimmed
- one tsp sea salt, divided
- one-eighth tsp freshly cracked black pepper

Directions:

1. Warm up the oven to 425 deg.F.
2. Stir the asparagus with half of salt and olive oil. At the base of a roasting tray, spread in a continuous sheet.
3. Season the salmon with salt and pepper. Place the asparagus on top of the skin-side down.

4. Lemon zest should be sprinkled over the asparagus, salmon, and lemon slices. Set them over the top.

5. Roast for around fifteen mins till the flesh of the fish is opaque, in the preheated oven.

Nutrition: Calories: 308; Fat: 18 gm; Carbs: 5 gm; Sugar: 2 gm; Fiber: 2 gm; Protein: 36 gm; Sodium: 542 mg

183. Orange and Maple-Glazed Salmon

Preparation Time: fifteen mins

Cooking Time: fifteen mins

Servings: two

Ingredients:

- 1 orange zest
- one tbsp low-sodium soy sauce
- 2 (4-6 oz.) salmon fillets, pin bones taken out
- 1 orange juice
- two tbsps pure maple syrup
- one tsp garlic powder

Directions:

1. Warm up the oven to 400 **deg.F.**

2. Set the orange juice and zest, soy sauce, maple syrup, and garlic powder in a little shallow container.

3. Place the salmon parts in the dish flesh-side down. Allow resting ten mins for marinating.

4. Put the salmon on a rimmed baking dish, skin-side up, and bake for fifteen mins, or till the flesh is opaque.

Nutrition: Calories: 297; Fat: 11; Carbs: 18 gm; Sugar: 15 gm; Fiber: 1 gm; Protein: 34 gm; Sodium: 528 mg

184. Cod with Ginger and Black Beans

Preparation Time: ten mins

Cooking Time: fifteen mins

Servings: two

Ingredients:

- 2 (6 oz.) cod fillets
- half tsp sea salt, divided
- 3 crushed garlic pieces
- two tbsps severed fresh cilantro leaves
- one tbsp extra-virgin olive oil
- half tbsp grated fresh ginger
- two tbsps freshly ground black pepper
- 1/2 (14 oz.) can black beans, drained

Directions:

1. Heat the olive oil in a big non-stick griddle or pan over medium-high heat till it starts shimmering.

2. Half of the salt, ginger, and pepper are used to season the fish. Cook for around four mins on all sides in the hot oil till the fish is opaque. Detach the cod from the pan and place it on a plate with aluminum foil tented over it.

3. Include the garlic to the griddle or pan and return it to the heat. Cook for thirty secs while continuously stirring.

4. Mix the black beans and the rest of the salt. Cook, stirring regularly, for five mins.

5. Include the cilantro and serve the black beans on top of the cod.

Nutrition: Calories: 419; Fat: 2 gm; Carbs: 33 gm; Sugar: 1 gm; Fiber: 8 gm; Protein: 50 gm; Sodium: 605 mg

185. Halibut Curry

Preparation Time: ten mins

Cooking Time: ten mins

Servings: two

Ingredients:

- one tsp ground turmeric
- 1-pound halibut, skin, and bones taken out, cut into one inch pieces
- 1/2 (14 oz.) can coconut milk
- one-eighth tsp ground black pepper
- one tbsp extra-virgin olive oil
- one tsp curry powder
- two teacups no-salt-added chicken broth
- quarter tsp sea salt

Directions:

1. Heat the olive oil in a non-stick griddle or pan over medium-high heat till it starts shimmering.

2. Include the curry powder and turmeric to a container. To bloom the spices, cook for two mins, stirring continuously.

3. Stir in halibut, coconut milk, chicken broth, pepper, and salt. Lower the heat to medium-low and bring to a simmer. Cook, stirring regularly, for six-seven mins, or till the fish is opaque.

Nutrition: Calories: 429; Fat: 47 gm; Carbs: 5 gm; Sugar: 1 gm; Fiber: 1 gm; Protein: 27 gm; Sodium: 507 mg

186. Chicken Cacciatore

Preparation Time: ten mins

Cooking Time: twenty mins

Servings: two

Ingredients:

- 1-pound skinless chicken, cut into bite-size pieces
- quarter teacup black olives, severed
- half tsp onion powder
- A tweak freshly ground black pepper
- one tbsp extra-virgin olive oil
- 1 (28 oz.) can crushed tomatoes, drained
- half tsp garlic powder
- quarter tsp sea salt

Directions:

1. Heat the olive oil in a non-stick griddle or pan over medium-high heat till it starts shimmering.
2. Cook till the chicken is browned.
3. Include the tomatoes, garlic powder, olives, salt, onion powder, and pepper, then stir to blend. Cook, stirring regularly, for ten mins.

Nutrition: Calories: 305; Fat: 11 gm; Carbs: 34 gm; Sugar: 23 gm; Fiber: 13 gm; Protein: 19 gm; Sodium: 1.171 mg

187. <u>Chicken and Bell Pepper Saute</u>

Preparation Time: five mins

Cooking Time: fifteen mins

Servings: two

Ingredients:

- 1 severed bell pepper
- 1-pound skinless chicken breasts, cut into bite-size pieces
- 1 ½ tablespoon extra-virgin olive oil
- 1/2 severed onion
- 3 crushed garlic pieces
- one-eighth tsp ground black pepper
- quarter tsp sea salt

Directions:

1. Heat the olive oil in a non-stick griddle or pan over medium-high heat till it starts shimmering.
2. Include the onion, red bell pepper, and chicken. Cook, stirring regularly, for ten mins.
3. Stir in the salt, garlic, and pepper inside a blending container. Cook for thirty secs while continuously stirring.

Nutrition: Calories: 179; Fat: 13 gm; Carbs: 6 gm; Sugar: 3 gm; Fiber: 1 gm; Protein: 10 gm; Sodium: 265 mg

188. <u>Chicken Salad Sandwiches</u>

Preparation Time: fifteen mins

Cooking Time: zero mins

Servings: two

Ingredients:

- two tbsps anti-inflammatory mayonnaise
- one tbsp severed fresh tarragon leaves
- one teacup chicken, severed, cooked, and skinless (from 1 rotisserie chicken)
- 1/2 crushed red bell pepper
- one tsp Dijon mustard
- 4 slices whole-wheat bread
- quarter tsp sea salt

Directions:

1. Blend the chicken, red bell pepper, mayonnaise, mustard, tarragon, and salt in a medium mixing container.
2. Spread on 2 pieces of bread and top it with the rest of the bread.

Nutrition: Calories: 315; Fat: 9 gm; Carbs: 30 gm; Sugar: 6 gm; Fiber: 4 gm; Protein: 28 gm; Sodium: 677 mg

189. <u>Rosemary Chicken</u>

Preparation Time: fifteen mins

Cooking Time: twenty mins

Servings: two

Ingredients:

- one tbsp extra-virgin olive oil
- 1-pound chicken breast tenders
- one tbsp severed fresh rosemary leaves
- one-eighth tsp ground black pepper
- quarter tsp sea salt

Directions:

1. Warm up the oven to 425 deg.F.
2. Set the chicken tenders on a baking sheet with a rim. Spray with salt, rosemary, and pepper after brushing them with olive oil.
3. For fifteen-twenty mins, keep in the oven, just prior to the juices run clear.

Nutrition: Calories: 389; Fat: 20 gm; Carbs: 1 gm; Sugar: 0 gm; Fiber: 1 gm; Protein: 49 gm; Sodium: 381 mg

190. <u>Gingered Turkey Meatballs</u>

Preparation Time: ten mins

Cooking Time: ten mins

Servings: two

Ingredients:

- half teacup shredded cabbage
- half tbsp grated fresh ginger
- half tsp onion powder
- 1-pound ground turkey
- two tbsps severed fresh cilantro leaves
- half tsp garlic powder
- quarter tsp sea salt
- one tbsp olive oil
- A tweak freshly ground black pepper

Directions:

1. Blend the cabbage, turkey, cilantro, ginger, onion powder, garlic powder, pepper, and salt in a big mixing container. Mix well. Make 10 (3/4 inch) meatballs out of the turkey mixture.
2. Heat the oil in a big non-stick griddle or pan over medium-high heat till it starts shimmering.
3. Cook for around ten mins, rotating the meatballs while they brown and you are done.

Nutrition: Calories: 408; Fat: 26 gm; Carbs: 4 gm; Sugar: 1 gm; Fiber: 1 gm; Protein: 47 gm; Sodium: 426 mg

191. <u>Turkey and Kale Saute</u>

Preparation Time: fifteen mins

Cooking Time: thirty-five mins

Servings: two

Ingredients:

- 1-pound ground turkey breast
- 1/2 severed onion
- half tsp sea salt
- 3 crushed garlic pieces
- one tbsp extra-virgin olive oil
- one teacup stemmed and severed kale
- one tbsp fresh thyme leaves
- A tweak freshly ground black pepper

Directions:

1. Heat the olive oil in a big non-stick griddle or pan over medium-high heat, till it starts shimmering.
2. Include the turkey, onion, kale, thyme, pepper, and salt. Cook, crumbling the turkey with a spoon till it browns, for around five mins.
3. Garlic can be included now. Cook for thirty mins while continuously stirring.

Nutrition: Calories: 413; Fat: 20 gm; Carbs: 7 gm; Sugar: 1 gm; Fiber: 1 gm; Protein: 50 gm; Sodium: 358 mg

192. Turkey with Bell Peppers and Rosemary

Preparation Time: fifteen mins

Cooking Time: ten mins

Servings: two

Ingredients:

- 1 severed red bell peppers
- one lb. boneless, skinless turkey breasts, cut into bite-size pieces
- quarter tsp sea salt
- 2 crushed garlic pieces
- two tbsps extra-virgin olive oil
- 1/2 severed onion
- one tbsp severed fresh rosemary leaves
- A tweak freshly ground black pepper

Directions:

1. Heat the olive oil in a non-stick griddle or pan over medium-high heat, till it starts shimmering.
2. Include the onion, red bell peppers, rosemary turkey, salt, and pepper. Cook till the turkey is cooked and the veggies are soft.
3. Garlic can be included now. Cook for an additional thirty secs.

Nutrition: Calories: 303; Fat: 14 gm; Carbs: 15 gm; Sugar: 10 gm; Fiber: 2 gm; Protein: 30 gm; Sodium: 387 mg

193. Mustard and Rosemary Pork Tenderloin

Preparation Time: fifteen mins

Cooking Time: fifteen mins

Servings: two

Ingredients:

- two tbsps Dijon mustard
- two tbsps fresh rosemary leaves
- quarter tsp sea salt
- 1/2 (one and half lbs.) pork tenderloin
- quarter teacup fresh parsley leaves
- 3 garlic pieces
- 1 ½ tablespoon extra-virgin olive oil
- one-eighth tsp ground black pepper

Directions:

1. Warm up the oven to 400 **deg.F.**
2. Blend the mustard, parsley, garlic, olive oil, rosemary, pepper, and salt in a blender or food processor. Pulse 20 times in 1-second intervals prior to a paste emerges. Rub the tenderloin with the paste and place it on a rimmed baking sheet.
3. Bake the pork for around fifteen mins or till an instant-read meat thermometer, reads 165 **deg.F.**
4. Allow resting for five mins prior to slicing and serving.

Nutrition: Calories: 362; Fat: 18 gm; Carbs: 5 gm; Sugar: 1 gm; Fiber: 2 gm; Protein: 2 gm; Sodium: 515 mg

194. Thin-Cut Pork Chops with Mustardy Kale

Preparation Time: ten mins

Cooking Time: twenty-five mins

Servings: two

Ingredients:

- one tsp sea salt, divided
- two tbsps Dijon mustard, divided
- 1/2 finely severed red onion
- one tbsp apple cider vinegar
- 2 thin-cut pork chops
- one-eighth tsp ground black pepper, divided
- 1 ½ tablespoon extra-virgin olive oil
- two teacups stemmed and severed kale

Directions:

1. Warm up the oven to 425 **deg.F.**
2. Half of salt and pepper are used to season the pork chops. Place them on a rimmed baking sheet and spread one tbsp of mustard over them. Bake for fifteen mins till an instant-read meat thermometer detects a temp. of 165 deg.F.
3. When the pork cooks, heat the olive oil in a big non-stick griddle or pan over medium-high heat till it starts shimmering.
4. Include the red onion and kale. Cook, stirring regularly, for around seven mins, or till the veggies soften.

5. Whisk together the rest of the tablespoon of mustard, the rest of the half salt, the cider vinegar, and the rest of the pepper in a wide mixing container. Toss with the kale. Cook for two mins, stirring occasionally.

Nutrition: Calories: 504; Fat: 39 gm; Carbs: 10 gm; Sugar: 1 gm; Fiber: 2 gm; Protein: 28 gm; Sodium: 755 mg

195. Beef Tenderloin with Savory Blueberry Sauce

Preparation Time: ten mins

Cooking Time: fifteen mins

Servings: two

Ingredients:

- one tsp sea salt, divided
- two tbsps extra-virgin olive oil
- quarter teacup tawny port
- 1 ½ tablespoon very cold butter, cut into pieces
- 2 beef tenderloin fillets, about 3⁄4 inch dense
- one-eighth tsp ground black pepper, divided
- 1 finely crushed shallot
- one teacup fresh blueberries

Directions:

1. Half salt and pepper are to be used to season the beef.
2. Heat the olive oil in a big griddle or pan over medium-high heat till it starts shimmering.
3. Include the seasoned steaks to the pan. Cook on all sides till an instant-read meat thermometer detects an internal temp. of 130 deg.F. Set aside on a plate of aluminum foil tented over it.
4. Get the griddle or pan back up to heat. Include the port, shallot, blueberries, and the rest of the salt and pepper to the pan. Scrape some browned pieces off the bottom of the griddle or pan with a wooden spoon. Set the heat to medium-low and bring to a simmer. Cook, stirring from time to time, and gently crush the blueberries for around 4 mins or till the liquid has reduced by half.
5. Set in the butter 1 slice at a time. Toss the meat back into the griddle or pan. Mix it once with the sauce to coat it. The rest of the sauce can be spooned over the meat prior to serving.

Nutrition: Calories: 554; Fat: 32 gm; Carbs: 14 gm; Sugar: 8 gm; Fiber: 2 gm; Protein: 50 gm; Sodium: 632 mg

196. Ground Beef Chili with Tomatoes

Preparation Time: ten mins

Cooking Time: fifteen mins

Servings: two

Ingredients:

- 1/2 severed onion
- 1 (14 oz.) can kidney beans, drained
- ½-pound extra-lean ground beef
- 1 (28 oz.) can severed tomatoes, undrained
- half tbsp chili powder
- quarter tsp sea salt
- half tsp garlic powder

Directions:

1. Cook the beef and onion in a big pot over medium-high heat for around five mins.
2. Include the kidney beans, tomatoes, garlic powder, chili powder, salt, and stir to blend. Bring to boil, then reduce to low heat.
3. Cook for ten mins, stirring occasionally.

Nutrition: Calories: 890; Fat: 20 gm; Carbs: 63 gm; Sugar: 13 gm; Fiber: 17 gm; Protein: 116 gm; Sodium: 562 mg

197. Fish Taco Salad with Strawberry Avocado Salsa

Preparation Time: twenty mins

Cooking Time: fifteen mins

Servings: two

Ingredients:

For the salsa:

- 2 hulled and cubed strawberries
- 1/2 cubed small shallot
- two tbsps finely severed fresh cilantro
- two tbsps freshly squeezed lime juice
- one-eighth tsp cayenne pepper
- 1/2 cubed avocado
- two tbsps canned black beans, rinsed and drained
- 1 thinly sliced green onions
- half tsp finely severed skinned ginger
- quarter tsp sea salt

For the fish salad:

- one tsp agave nectar
- two teacups arugula
- one tbsp extra-virgin olive or avocado oil
- half tbsp freshly squeezed lime juice
- 1-pound light fish (halibut, cod, or red snapper), cut into 2 fillets
- quarter tsp ground black pepper
- half tsp sea salt

Directions:

For the salsa:

1. Warm up the grill, whether it's gas or charcoal.
2. Include the avocado, beans, strawberries, shallot, cilantro, green onions, salt, ginger, lime juice, and cayenne pepper in a medium mixing cup. Put aside after mixing till all the components are well blended.

For the fish salad:

1. Whisk the agave, oil, and lime juice in a small container. Set the arugula with the vinaigrette in a big mixing container.

2. Season the fish fillets with pepper and salt. Grill the fish for seven-nine mins over direct high heat, flipping once during cooking. The fish should be translucent and quickly flake.

3. Place one teacup of arugula salad on each plate to eat. Cover each salad with a fillet and a heaping spoonful of salsa.

Nutrition: Calories: 878; Fat: 26 gm; Carbs: 53 gm; Sugar: 15 gm; Fiber: 18 gm; Protein: 119 gm; Sodium: 582 mg

198. **Beef and Bell Pepper Stir-Fry**

Preparation Time: five mins

Cooking Time: ten mins

Servings: two

Ingredients:

- 3 scallions, white and green parts, severed
- one tbsp grated fresh ginger
- 2 crushed garlic pieces
- ½-pound extra-lean ground beef
- 1 severed red bell peppers
- quarter tsp sea salt

Directions:

1. Cook the beef for around five mins in a big non-stick griddle or pan till it browns.

2. Include the scallions, ginger, red bell peppers, and salt. Cook, stirring occasionally, for around four mins or till the bell peppers are tender.

3. Garlic can be included now. Cook for thirty secs while continuously stirring. Switch off the flame, and you are done.

Nutrition: Calories: 599; Fat: 19 gm; Carbs: 9 gm; Sugar: 4 gm; Fiber: 2 gm; Protein: 97 gm; Sodium: 520 mg

199. **Veggie Pizza with Cauliflower-Yam Crust**

Preparation Time: five mins

Cooking Time: one hr ten mins

Servings: two

Ingredients:

- half medium skinned and severed garnet yam
- one tsp sea salt, divided
- half tbsp coconut oil, plus more for greasing pizza stone
- quarter teacup sliced cremini mushrooms
- 1/4 medium head cauliflower, cut into small florets
- half tbsp dried Italian herbs
- half teacup flour brown rice
- 1/2 sliced small red onion
- 1/2 zucchini or yellow summer squash
- two tbsps vegan pesto
- half teacup spinach

Directions:

1. Heat the oven to 400 **deg.**F or preheat the pizza stone in case you have one.

2. Set a big pot with 1 inch of water, place a steamer basket. Put the yam and cauliflower in the steamer basket and steam for fifteen mins, or till both are quickly pricked with a fork. If you overcook the vegetables, they can get too soggy.

3. Place the vegetables in a food blender or processor and pulse till smooth. Blend in the Italian herbs and half a teaspoon of salt till smooth. Set the mixture in a big mixing container. Gradually whisk in the flour till it is well mixed.

4. Use coconut oil to grease the pizza stone or a pizza plate. In the middle of the pizza stone, pile the cauliflower mixture. Spread the pizza dough uniformly roundly or circularly (much like frosting) with a spatula till the crust is around 1/8 inches dense.

5. Bake for around forty-five mins. To get the top crispy, switch on the broiler and cook it for two mins.

6. In a medium griddle or pan, melt the coconut oil at middling temp. Cook for two mins after adding the onion. Include the squash, mushrooms, and the rest of the components to a big blending container. Saute for three to four mins with a quarter teaspoon of salt. Detach the spinach from the heat when it starts to wilt.

7. Evenly, plate the pesto around the pizza crust. Over the pesto, spread the sautéed vegetables. It's time to slice the pizza and eat it.

Nutrition: Calories: 329; Fat: 17 gm; Carbs: 9 gm; Sugar: 3 gm; Fiber: 5 gm; Protein: 37 gm; Sodium: 430 mg

200. **Toasted Pecan Quinoa Burgers**

Preparation Time: five mins

Cooking Time: thirty mins

Servings: two

Ingredients:

- two teacups vegetable broth, divided
- one tsp sea salt
- two tbsps sesame seeds
- half tsp dried oregano
- quarter teacup canned black beans,
- two tbsps pecans
- half teacup quinoa, rinsed and drained
- quarter teacup sunflower seeds
- half tsp ground cumin
- 1/2 shredded carrot
- Freshly ground black pepper
- 1/2 thinly sliced avocado
- half tsp coconut or sunflower oil

Directions:

1. Warm up the oven to 375 deg.F.

2. Roast the pecans for five-seven mins on a baking sheet.

3. In a big saucepan, bring one teacup of broth, quinoa, and salt to a boil at medium-high temp. Set the heat to a minimum, cover, and cook for twenty mins, stirring occasionally.

4. Inside a blending container, grind the pecans, cumin, sesame seeds, sunflower seeds, and oregano to a medium-coarse texture.

5. Combine a half cup of quinoa, carrots, nuts, and beans in a large container. Slowly pour the remaining cup of broth while stirring until the paste becomes sticky. Season with salt and pepper to taste.

6. Set the mixture into 2 (1/2-inch dense) patties and cook, put in the fridge them immediately.

7. Melt coconut oil in a large griddle or pan on medium-high heat. Cook for two mins per side. Repeat for the remaining patties. Avocado slices can top burgers.

Nutrition:
Calories: 432; Fat: 12 gm; Carbs: 12 gm; Sugar: 5 gm; Fiber: 3 gm; Protein: 57 gm; Sodium: 566 mg

201. Sizzling Salmon and Quinoa

Preparation Time: ten mins

Cooking Time: thirty mins

Servings: two

Ingredients:

- half tsp extra-virgin olive oil
- half teacup quinoa, rinsed and drained
- 1/4 pound sliced chanterelle mushrooms
- half teacup frozen small peas
- one tbsp severed fresh basil
- 1 head garlic
- one and half teacups mushroom broth, divided
- one tbsp coconut oil
- half teacup shredded brussels sprouts
- one tbsp nutritional yeast
- half tbsp dried oregano
- Sea salt and freshly ground black pepper
- ¼-pound salmon, skin, and bones taken out, cut into one inch cubes

Directions:

1. Warm up the oven to 350 **deg.F.**

2. Detach the top of the garlic head to reveal the pieces. Cover the head in foil; drizzle with olive oil. Set in the oven for fifty mins to roast.

3. Mix quinoa and one teacup of broth in a large saucepan. Boil over high heat, then lower to low, cover, and simmer without stirring for twenty mins. Use a quarter teacup of quinoa for this dish, saving the rest.

4. Heat the coconut oil in a big griddle or pan at middling temp. Saute for five mins, or prior to the mushrooms release liquid and become tender.

5. Cook brussels sprouts for three mins, adding quarter cup broth if needed to prevent sticking.

6. Saute for five mins, stirring regularly, with the peas, basil, nutritional yeast, and oregano.

7. Mix the salmon in the pan. Gently squeeze garlic into it. Cook, covered, for four–five mins, stirring occasionally.

8. Mix the remaining quarter cup broth and quarter cup quinoa in the griddle or pan until fully combined. Use pepper and salt as needed.

9. Serve.

Nutrition: Calories: 599; Fat: 20 gm; Carbs: 10 gm; Sugar: 4 gm; Fiber: 6 gm; Protein: 88 gm; Sodium: 662 mg

Breakfast

202. Mango Ginger Smoothie

Preparation Time: five mins

Servings: one

Ingredients:

- half teacup red lentils, cooked cooled
- one teacup mango chunks, frozen
- three-quarter teacup carrot juice
- one tsp fresh ginger, severed
- one tsp honey
- 1 tweak ground cardamom
- 3 Ice cubes

Directions:

1. Include all components into the blender and blend on high, about two to three mins.
2. Garnish with cardamom.

Nutrition: Calories: 352; Carbohydrates: 78.9 gm; Fats: 1.1 gm; Proteins: 12.3 gm; Fiber: 9.6 gm

203. Cherry Spinach Smoothie

Preparation Time: five mins

Servings: one

Ingredients:

- one teacup kefir, low-fat
- one teacup frozen cherries
- half teacup baby spinach leaves
- quarter teacup avocado, mashed
- one tbsp salted almond butter
- ½-inch piece ginger, skinned
- one tsp chia seeds

Directions:

1. Include all components into the blender and blend on high, about two to three mins.
2. Pour smoothie into the glass.
3. Garnish with chia seeds.

Nutrition: Calories: 410; Carbohydrates: 46.6 gm; Fats: 20.1 gm; Proteins: 17.4 gm; Fiber: 10.1 gm

204. Banana Cacao Smoothie

Preparation Time: five mins

Servings: two

Ingredients:

- 2 frozen bananas, sliced
- quarter teacup cacao bliss
- quarter teacup almond butter
- two tbsps hemp hearts
- two teacups non-dairy milk
- half teacup ice

Directions:

1. Include all components into the blender and blend on high, about two to three mins.
2. Pour smoothie into the glass.

Nutrition: Calories: 515; Carbohydrates: 48 gm; Fats: 31 gm; Proteins: 22 gm; Fiber: 11 gm

205. Spinach and Egg Scramble with Raspberries

Preparation Time: ten mins

Cooking time: five mins

Servings: one

Ingredients:

- one tsp canola oil
- one and half teacups baby spinach
- 2 eggs, beaten
- A tweak Kosher salt
- A tweak ground pepper
- 1 slice whole-grain bread, toasted
- half teacup fresh raspberries

Directions:

1. Include oil into the griddle and heat it over medium-high flame.
2. Include spinach and cook for one to two mins till wilted.
3. Transfer the spinach to the medium plate.
4. Clean the pan and put it at medium flame. Then, include eggs and cook for one to two mins.
5. Include pepper, salt, and spinach and stir well.
6. Top with raspberries. Serve with toasted bread.

Nutrition: Calories: 296; Carbohydrates: 20.9 gm; Fats: 15.7 gm; Proteins: 17.8 gm; Fiber: 7 gm

206. Blackberry Smoothie

Preparation Time: five mins

Servings: one

Ingredients:

- one teacup fresh blackberries
- ½ banana
- half teacup plain whole-milk Greek yogurt
- one tbsp honey
- one and half tsps fresh lemon juice
- one tsp fresh ginger, severed

Directions:

1. Include all components into the blender and blend on high, about two to three mins.
2. Pour smoothie into the glass.

Nutrition: Calories: 316; Carbohydrates: 53 gm; Fats: 7 gm; Proteins: 15 gm; Fiber: 10 gm

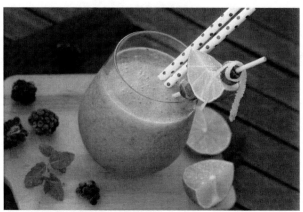

207. Veggie Frittata

Preparation Time: five mins

Cooking Time: ten mins

Servings: one

Ingredients:

- one tbsp canola oil
- 2 scallions, green and white parts separated, thinly sliced
- Mixed veggies – one teacup carrots, broccoli, and cauliflower, severed
- one-eighth tsp salt
- 2 eggs, beaten
- two tbsps cheddar cheese, shredded
- 1 orange, cut into wedges

Directions:

1. Include oil into a griddle and put it at medium-high flame.
2. Include salt, veggies, and whites scallions and cook for three to five mins till browned. Include green scallions and stir well.
3. Pour eggs over the vegetables and sprinkle with cheese.
4. Cover with a foil and take out from the flame.
5. Let sit for four to five mins.
6. Serve with orange wedges.

Nutrition: Calories: 491; Carbohydrates: 37 gm; Fats: 29 gm; Proteins: 22 gm; Fiber: 7 gm

208. Chocolate Banana Protein Smoothie

Preparation Time: five mins

Servings: one

Ingredients:

- 1 banana, frozen
- half teacup red lentils, cooked
- half teacup milk, non-fat
- two tsps unsweetened cocoa powder
- one tsp pure maple syrup

Directions:

1. Mix the syrup, cocoa, milk, lentils, and banana into the blender and blend till smooth.
2. Serve!

Nutrition: Calories: 310; Carbohydrates: 63.8 gm; Fats: 1.8 gm; Proteins: 15.3 gm; Fiber: 8.5 gm

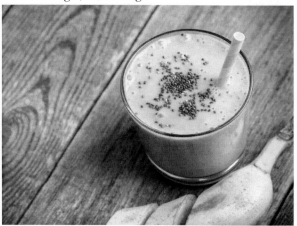

209. Cocoa Almond French toast

Preparation Time: ten mins

Cooking time: six mins

Servings: two

Ingredients:

- half teacup unsweetened almond milk
- 1 egg
- half tsp ground cinnamon
- half tsp ground nutmeg
- quarter teacup almond, severed
- Non-stick cooking spray
- 4 slices whole wheat bread
- two tbsps chocolate syrup, sugar-free
- quarter teacup raspberries

Directions:

1. Include nutmeg, cinnamon, eggs, and almond milk into the dish and keep ½ tablespoon of severed almonds to garnish.
2. Place rest of the severed almonds in another container.
3. Let coat the griddle with a cooking spray.
4. Heat the griddle over medium flame.
5. Meanwhile, immerse each bread slice into the egg mixture.
6. Then, dip soaked bread in the almonds and coat on both sides.
7. Place coated bread slices onto the griddle and cook for four to six mins till golden brown.
8. Cut bread in half, lengthwise. Place onto the two serving plates.
9. Spray with chocolate syrup.

10. Top with raspberries and severed almonds.

Nutrition:

Calories: 250; Carbohydrates: 28.6 gm; Fats: 11.7 gm; Proteins: 15 gm; Fiber: 7.9 gm

210. Muesli with Raspberries

Preparation Time: five mins

Servings: one

Ingredients:

- one-third teacup muesli
- one teacup raspberries
- three-quarter teacup milk, low-fat

Directions:

1. Place muesli into the container. Top with raspberries.
2. Serve with warm or cold water.

Nutrition: Calories: 288; Carbohydrates: 51.8 gm; Fats: 6.6 gm; Proteins: 13 gm; Fiber: 13.3 gm

211. Mocha Overnight Oats

Preparation Time: ten mins

Chill time: eight hrs

Servings: one

Ingredients:

- half teacup rolled oats
- half teacup milk, low fat
- quarter teacup cooled coffee
- one tbsp pure maple syrup
- one and half tsps chia seeds
- one and half tsps cocoa powder
- one tbsp walnuts, toasted, severed
- one tsp cacao nibs

Directions:

1. Combine cocoa powder, chia seeds, maple syrup, coffee, milk, and oats in a container. Put it in the fridge overnight or for eight hrs with a lid.
2. Top with cacao nibs and walnuts.

Nutrition: Calories: 379; Carbohydrates: 53 gm; Fats: 15.1 gm; Proteins: 12.6 gm; Fiber: 9.1 gm

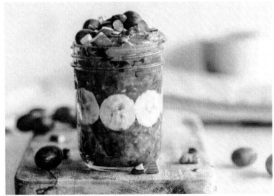

212. Baked Banana-Nut Oatmeal Cups

Preparation Time: ten mins

Baking time: twenty-five mins

Servings: twelve

Ingredients:

- three teacups rolled oats
- one and half teacups low-fat milk
- 2 bananas, mashed
- one-third teacup brown sugar
- 2 eggs, beaten
- one tsp baking powder
- one tsp ground cinnamon
- one tsp vanilla extract
- half tsp salt
- half teacup pecans, severed, toasted

Directions:

1. Warm up the oven to 375 deg.F.
2. Let coat the muffin tin with cooking spray.
3. Mix the salt, vanilla, cinnamon, baking powder, eggs, brown sugar, bananas, milk, and oats into the container.
4. Fold in the pecans. Place mixture into the muffin cups and bake for twenty-five mins.
5. Let cool it for ten mins.
6. Serve and relish!

Nutrition: Calories: 176; Carbohydrates: 26.4 gm; Protein: 5.2 gm; Fat: 6.2 gm; Fiber: 3.1 gm

213. Pineapple Green Smoothie

Preparation Time: five mins

Servings: one

Ingredients:

- half teacup unsweetened almond milk
- one-third teacup plain Greek yogurt, non-fat
- one teacup baby spinach
- one teacup frozen banana slices
- half teacup frozen pineapple chunks
- one tbsp chia seeds
- one to two tsps pure maple syrup or honey

Directions:

1. Include yogurt and almond milk into the blender and blend till smooth.
2. Then, include spinach, pineapple, bananas, honey, or maple syrup, and chia into the blender and blend till smooth.
3. Serve and relish!

Nutrition: Calories: 297; Carbohydrates: 54.3 gm; Protein: 12.8 gm; Fat: 5.7 gm; Fiber: 9.8 gm

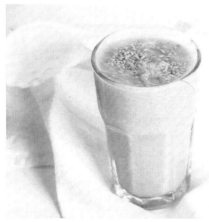

214. Pumpkin Bread

Preparation Time: ten mins

Cooking Time: one hr fifteen mins

Servings: twelve

Ingredients:

- 5 tablespoons water
- two tbsps flaxseed meal
- three-quarter teacup unsweetened almond milk
- three-quarter teacup sugar
- one-third teacup canola oil
- one tsp vanilla extract
- one and half teacups unseasoned pumpkin puree
- two teacups white whole-wheat flour
- two tsps baking powder
- one tsp pumpkin pie spice or cinnamon
- half tsp salt
- half teacup bittersweet chocolate chips

Directions:

1. Warm up the oven to 350 deg.F.
2. Let coat the loaf pan with cooking spray.
3. Mix the flaxseed meal and water into the container. Let sit for a couple of mins.
4. Whisk the flaxseed mixture, vanilla, oil, sugar, and almond milk into the container. Then, include pumpkin puree and stir well.
5. Whisk the salt, pumpkin pie spice, flour, and baking powder into the container. Include wet components; stir well.
6. Include chocolate chips and stir well.
7. Transfer the batter to the pan. Bake for one hour and fifteen mins.
8. Let cool it for one hour.
9. Serve and relish!

Nutrition: Calories: 191; Carbohydrates: 30.5 gm; Protein: 3.3 gm; Fat: 7 gm; Fiber: 3.3 gm

215. Banana-Bran Muffins

Preparation Time: ten mins

Cooking Time: twenty-five mins

Servings: twelve

Ingredients:

- 2 eggs
- two-third teacup brown sugar
- one teacup ripe bananas, mashed
- one teacup buttermilk
- one teacup unprocessed wheat bran
- quarter teacup canola oil
- one tsp vanilla extract
- one teacup whole-wheat flour
- three-quarter teacup all-purpose flour
- one and half tsps baking powder
- half tsp baking soda
- half tsp ground cinnamon
- quarter tsp salt
- half teacup chocolate chips
- one-third teacup walnuts, severed

Directions:

1. Warm up the oven to 400 deg.F.
2. Let coat twelve muffin cups with cooking spray.
3. Whisk the brown sugar and eggs into the container till smooth.
4. Include vanilla, oil, wheat bran, buttermilk, and bananas and whisk it well.
5. Whisk the salt, cinnamon, baking soda, baking powder, flour, all-purpose flour, and whole-wheat flour into the container.
6. Make a well in the middle of the dry components and then include wet components and stir well.
7. Include chocolate chips and stir well. Place batter into the muffin cups and sprinkle with walnuts. Bake it for fifteen to twenty-five mins till golden brown.
8. Let cool it for five mins.
9. Serve and relish!

Nutrition: Calories: 200; Carbohydrates: 34.1 gm; Protein: 4.8 gm; Fat: 7 gm; Fiber: 3.9 gm

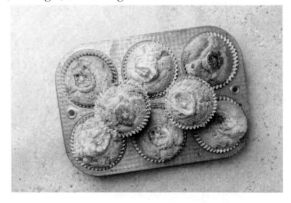

216. Banana Bread

Preparation Time: fifteen mins

Cooking Time: one hr

Servings: ten

Ingredients:

- one and three-quarter teacups white whole-wheat flour
- one and half tsps baking powder
- one tsp ground cinnamon
- half tsp salt
- quarter tsp baking soda
- three-quarter teacup sugar
- quarter teacup unsalted butter or coconut oil, softened
- 2 eggs
- one and half teacups ripe bananas, mashed
- quarter teacup buttermilk
- one tsp vanilla extract
- half teacup walnuts or chocolate chips, severed

Directions:

1. Warm up the oven to 350 deg.F.
2. Let coat the loaf pan with cooking spray.
3. Whisk the baking soda, salt, cinnamon, flour, and baking powder into the container.
4. Include butter and sugar into the container and beat it well using an electric mixer at medium-high temp.
5. Include eggs and beat it well. Include flour mixture and beat on low speed and then fold in chocolate chips or walnuts.
6. Place batter into the pan. Bake for forty-five to fifty-five mins.
7. Serve and relish!

Nutrition: Calories: 221; Carbohydrates: 39.4 gm; Protein: 4.7 gm; Fat: 5.9 gm; Fiber: 3.1 gm

217. Chocolate-Raspberry Oatmeal

Preparation Time: ten mins

Cooking time: five-seven mins

Servings: four

Ingredients:

- one and half teacups regular rolled oats
- two tbsps unsweetened cocoa powder
- quarter tsp salt
- three teacups unsweetened almond milk
- one teacup fresh red raspberries
- 4 teaspoon chocolate syrup

Directions:

1. Pour salt, cocoa powder, and oats into the saucepan. Add almond milk and mix well. Boil on medium heat. Lower the heat and simmer five–seven mins.

2. Take out from the flame. Let stand for two mins.
3. Place oatmeal mixture into the serving bowls.
4. Top with quarter teacup of raspberries.
5. Spray with one teaspoon chocolate syrup.

Nutrition: Calories: 157; Carbohydrates: 26.2 gm; Protein: 5.4 gm; Fat: 4.7 gm; Fiber: 6.6 gm

218. Chai Chia Pudding

Preparation Time: ten mins

Chill time: eight hrs

Servings: one

Ingredients:

- half teacup unsweetened almond milk
- two tbsps chia seeds
- two tsps pure maple syrup
- quarter tsp vanilla extract
- quarter tsp ground cinnamon
- Pinch of ground cardamom
- Pinch of ground pieces
- half teacup banana, sliced
- one tbsp unsalted pistachios, severed, roasted

Directions:

1. Include pieces, cardamom, cinnamon, vanilla, maple syrup, chia, and almond milk into the container and stir well.
2. Cover with a lid and place it into the fridge for eight hours.
3. When ready to serve, blend it well. Place half of the pudding into the glass and top with half of pistachios and bananas.
4. Then, include the rest of the pudding and top with rest of the pistachios and bananas.
5. Serve and relish!

Nutrition: Calories: 264; Carbohydrates: 38.2 gm; Protein: 6.3 gm; Fat: 11.2 gm; Fiber: 10.8 gm

219. Apple Cinnamon Oatmeal

Preparation Time: five mins

Cooking Time: forty mins

Servings: four

Ingredients:

- 4 crisp apples
- one teacup steel-cut oats
- four teacups water
- three tbsps brown sugar
- half tsp ground cinnamon
- quarter tsp salt
- half teacup nonfat plain greek yogurt

Directions:

1. Firstly, cut two apples with a box grater.

2. Include oats into the saucepan and cook at medium-high flame till toasted, for two mins.

3. Then, include shredded apples and water and boil it.

4. Then, lower the heat and cook for ten mins.

5. During this, chop two apples.

6. Add salt, cinnamon, two tablespoons brown sugar, and diced apples to cooked oats. Stir thoroughly for fifteen-twenty mins.

7. Place between four bowls.

8. Top with ¾ teaspoon brown sugar and two tablespoons of yogurt.

Nutrition: Calories: 282; Carbohydrates: 59.1 gm; Protein: 8 gm; Fat: 2.7 gm; Fiber: 6.3 gm

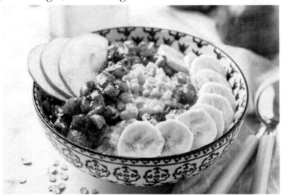

220. **Apple Butter Bran Muffins**

Preparation Time: five mins

Cooking Time: forty mins

Servings: twelve

Ingredients:

- half teacup raisins
- three-quarter teacup whole-wheat flour
- three-quarter teacup all-purpose flour
- two and half tsps baking powder
- quarter tsp salt
- half tsp ground cinnamon
- three-quarter teacup unprocessed wheat bran
- 1 egg, beaten
- half teacup low-fat milk
- half teacup spiced apple butter
- half teacup brown sugar
- quarter teacup canola oil
- three tbsps molasses
- one teacup apple, cubed, skinned

Directions:

1. Warm up the oven to 375 deg.F.

2. Let coat twelve muffin cups with cooking spray.

3. Include raisins into the container and cover with hot water and keep it aside.

4. Mix cinnamon, salt, baking powder, flour, all-purpose flour, and whole-wheat flour in the container. Add bran and mix well.

5. Mix molasses, oil, brown sugar, apple butter, egg, and milk in the container. Create a dry well and place in wet. Drain and add raisins to apple cubes. Thoroughly stir.

6. Place batter into the pan. Bake for eighteen to twenty-two mins.

7. Let cool the pan for five mins.

8. Serve and relish!

Nutrition: Calories: 204; Carbohydrates: 37.6 gm; Protein: 3.9 gm; Fat: 5.7 gm; Fiber: 3.7 gm

221. **Pineapple Raspberry Parfaits**

Preparation Time: five mins

Servings: four

Ingredients:

- two teacups nonfat peach yogurt
- ½ pint raspberries
- one and half teacups pineapple chunks

Directions:

1. Place pineapple, raspberries, and yogurt into the four glasses.

2. Serve and relish!

Nutrition: Calories: 155; Carbohydrates: 33 gm; Protein: 5.7 gm; Fat: 0.5 gm; Fiber: 2.9 gm

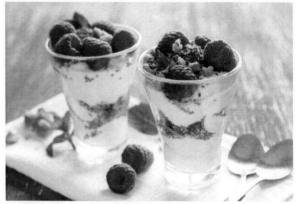

222. **Berry Chia Pudding**

Preparation Time: five mins

Chill time: eight hrs

Servings: two

Ingredients:

- one and three-quarter teacups blackberries, raspberries, or cubed mango
- one teacup unsweetened almond milk
- quarter teacup chia seeds
- one tbsp pure maple syrup
- ¾ teaspoon vanilla extract
- half teacup whole-milk plain greek yogurt
- quarter teacup granola

Directions:

1. Include milk and one and quarter teacups fruit into the blender and blend till smooth.
2. Transfer it to the medium container. Include vanilla, syrup, and chia and blend well. Place it into the fridge for eight hours.
3. Place pudding into the two bowls. Layering each serving with two tablespoons of granola, quarter teacup yogurt, and the rest of the quarter teacup of fruit.
4. Serve!

Nutrition: Calories: 343; Carbohydrates: 39.4 gm; Protein: 13.8 gm; Fat: 15.4 gm; Fiber: 14.9 gm

223. Spinach Avocado Smoothie

Preparation Time: five mins

Servings: one

Ingredients:

- one teacup nonfat plain yogurt
- one teacup fresh spinach
- 1 banana, frozen
- ¼ avocado
- two tbsps water
- one tsp honey

Directions:

1. Mix the honey, water, avocado, banana, spinach, and yogurt into the blender and blend till smooth.
2. Serve and relish!

Nutrition: Calories: 357; Carbohydrates: 57.8 gm; Protein: 17.7 gm; Fat: 8.2 gm; Fiber: 7.8 gm

224. Strawberry Pineapple Smoothie

Preparation Time: five mins

Servings: one

Ingredients:

- one teacup frozen strawberries
- one teacup fresh pineapple, severed
- three-quarter teacup unsweetened almond milk, chilled
- one tbsp almond butter

Directions:

1. Mix the almond butter, almond milk, pineapple, and strawberries into the blender and process till smooth.
2. Include almond milk more if required.
3. Serve and relish!

Nutrition:

Calories: 255; Carbohydrates: 39 gm; Protein: 5.6 gm; Fat: 11.1 gm; Fiber: 7.8 gm

225. Peach Blueberry Parfaits

Preparation Time: ten mins

Servings: two

Ingredients:

- 6-ounce vanilla, peach or blueberry fat-free yogurt
- one teacup sweetener multigrain clusters cereal
- 1 peach, pitted and sliced
- half teacup fresh blueberries
- quarter tsp ground cinnamon

Directions:

1. Include half of the yogurt into the two glasses.
2. Top with half of the cereal. Top with half of cinnamon, blueberries, and peaches. Place rest of the blueberries, peaches, cereal, and yogurt.
3. Serve and relish!

Nutrition: Calories: 166; Carbohydrates: 34 gm; Protein: 11 gm; Fat: 1 gm; Fiber: 7 gm

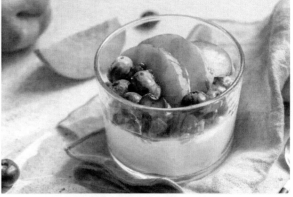

226. Raspberry Yogurt Cereal Bowl

Preparation Time: five mins

Servings: one

Ingredients:

- one teacup nonfat plain yogurt
- half teacup, shredded wheat cereal
- quarter teacup fresh raspberries
- two tsps mini chocolate chips
- one tsp pumpkin seeds
- quarter tsp ground cinnamon

Directions:

1. Include yogurt into the container.
2. Top with cinnamon, pumpkin seeds, chocolate chips, raspberries, and shredded wheat.
3. Serve and relish!

Nutrition:

Calories: 290; Carbohydrates: 47.8 gm; Protein: 18.4 gm; Fat: 4.6 gm; Fiber: 6 gm

227. Avocado toast

Preparation Time: ten mins

Servings: one

Ingredients:

- one teacup mixed salad greens
- one tsp red-wine vinegar

- one tsp extra-virgin olive oil
- Pinch of salt
- Pinch of pepper
- 2 slices sprouted whole-wheat bread, toasted
- quarter teacup plain hummus
- quarter teacup alfalfa sprouts
- ¼ avocado, sliced
- two tsps unsalted sunflower seeds

Directions:
1. Firstly, toss greens with pepper, salt, oil, and vinegar into the container.
2. Spread each slice of toast with two tablespoons of hummus and top with greens, sprouts, avocado, and spinach.
3. Spray with sunflower seeds.
4. Serve and relish!

Nutrition:
Calories: 429; Carbohydrates: 46.4 gm; Protein: 16.2 gm; Fat: 21.9 gm; Fiber: 15.1 gm

228. Loaded Pita Pockets

Preparation Time: five mins

Servings: one

Ingredients:

- 1 whole wheat pita bread, halved
- half teacup low-fat Cottage cheese
- 4 walnut halves, severed
- 1 banana, sliced

Directions:
1. Fill each pita with banana, walnuts, and cottage cheese.

Nutrition: Calories: 307; Carbohydrates: 46 gm; Protein: 21 gm; Fat: 8.5 gm; Fiber: 11 gm

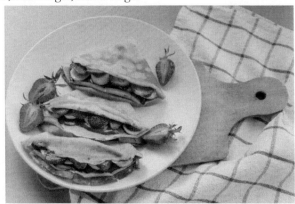

229. Pear Pancakes

Preparation Time: ten mins

Cooking Time: twenty mins

Servings: four

Ingredients:

- one teacup whole wheat flour

- quarter tsp baking soda
- quarter tsp baking powder
- one teacup pears
- 2 eggs
- one teacup milk

Directions:
2. In a container, blend all components and mix well.
3. In a griddle, heat olive oil.
4. Pour ¼ of the batter and cook each pancake for one-two mins on all sides.
5. When ready, take out from heat and serve.

Nutrition: Calories 277; Fat 19 gm; Carbohydrates 56 gm; Protein 13.8 gm

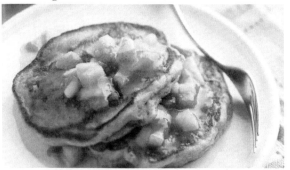

230. Almond Pancakes

Preparation Time: ten mins

Cooking Time: thirty mins

Servings: four

Ingredients:

- one teacup whole wheat flour
- quarter tsp baking soda
- quarter tsp baking powder
- one teacup almonds
- 2 eggs
- one teacup milk

Directions:
1. In a container, blend all components and mix well.
2. In a griddle, heat olive oil.
3. Pour ¼ of the batter and cook each pancake for one-two mins on all sides.
4. When ready, take out from heat and serve.

Nutrition: Calories 234; Fat 20 gm; Carbohydrates 4.0 gm; Protein 10 gm

231. Avocado Pancakes

Preparation Time: ten mins

Cooking Time: twenty mins

Servings: four

Ingredients:

- one teacup whole wheat flour
- quarter tsp baking soda

- quarter tsp baking powder
- 2 eggs
- one teacup milk
- 1cup mashed avocado

Directions:

1. In a container, blend all components and mix well.
2. In a griddle, heat olive oil.
3. Pour ¼ of the batter and cook each pancake for one-two mins on all sides.
4. When ready, take out from heat and serve.

Nutrition:

Calories 310; Fat 18 gm; Carbohydrates 34 gm; Protein 7 gm

232. Strawberry Pancakes

Preparation Time: ten mins

Cooking Time: twenty mins

Servings: four

Ingredients:

- one teacup whole wheat flour
- quarter tsp baking soda
- quarter tsp baking powder
- one teacup strawberries
- 2 eggs
- one teacup milk

Directions:

1. In a container, blend all components and mix well.
2. In a griddle, heat olive oil.
3. Pour ¼ of the batter and cook each pancake for one-two mins on all sides.
4. When ready, take out from heat and serve.

Nutrition: Calories 102; Fat 4.7 gm; Carbohydrates 12 gm; Protein 3 gm

233. Carambola Pancakes

Preparation Time: ten mins

Cooking Time: thirty mins

Servings: four

Ingredients:

- one teacup whole wheat flour
- quarter tsp baking soda
- quarter tsp baking powder
- 2 eggs
- one teacup milk
- one teacup carambola

Directions:

1. In a container, blend all components and mix well.
2. In a griddle, heat olive oil.
3. Pour ¼ of the batter and cook each pancake for one-two mins on all sides.
4. When ready, take out from heat and serve.

Nutrition: Calories 774; Fat 35 gm; Carbohydrates 108 gm; Protein 5.89 gm

234. Ginger Muffins

Preparation Time: ten mins

Cooking Time: twenty mins

Servings: eight-twelve

Ingredients:

- 2 eggs
- one tbsp olive oil
- one teacup milk
- two teacups whole wheat flour
- one tsp baking soda
- quarter tsp baking soda
- one tsp ginger
- one tsp cinnamon
- quarter teacup molasses

Directions:

1. In a container, blend all wet components.
2. In another container, blend all dry components.
3. Blend wet and dry components.
4. Fold in ginger and mix well.
5. Pour mixture into 8-12 prepared muffin cups, fill 2/3 of the cups.
6. Bake for eighteen-twenty mins at 375 F.
7. When ready, take out from the oven and serve.

Nutrition: Calories 18707; Fat 6.4 gm; Carbohydrates 29.0 gm; Protein 6.1 gm

235. Carrot Muffins

Preparation Time: ten mins

Cooking Time: twenty mins

Servings: eight-twelve

Ingredients:

- 2 eggs
- one tbsp olive oil
- one teacup milk
- two teacups whole wheat flour
- one tsp baking soda
- quarter tsp baking soda
- one tsp cinnamon
- one teacup carrots

Directions:

1. In a container, blend all wet components.
2. In another container, blend all dry components.
3. Blend wet and dry components.
4. Pour mixture into 8-12 prepared muffin cups, fill 2/3 of the cups.
5. Bake for eighteen-twenty mins at 375 deg.F.
6. When ready, take out from the oven and serve.

Nutrition: Calories 342; Fat 12.89 gm; Carbohydrates 50.3 gm; Protein 6.85 gm

236. Blueberry Muffins

Preparation Time: ten mins

Cooking Time: twenty mins

Servings: eight-twelve mins

Ingredients:

- 2 eggs
- one tbsp olive oil
- one teacup milk
- two teacups whole wheat flour
- one tsp baking soda
- quarter tsp baking soda
- one tsp cinnamon
- one teacup blueberries

Directions:

1. In a container, blend all wet components.
2. In another container, blend all dry components.
3. Blend wet and dry components.
4. Fold in blueberries and mix well.
5. Pour mixture into 8-12 prepared muffin cups, fill 2/3 of the cups.
6. Bake for eighteen-twenty mins at 375 deg.F, when ready take out, and serve.

Nutrition: Calories 467; Fat 13 gm; Carbohydrates 68 gm; Protein 6 gm

237. Coconut Muffins

Preparation Time: ten mins

Cooking Time: twenty mins

Servings: eight-twelve

Ingredients:

- 2 eggs
- one tbsp olive oil
- one teacup milk
- two teacups whole wheat flour
- one tsp baking soda
- quarter tsp baking soda
- one tsp cinnamon
- one teacup coconut flakes

Directions:

1. In a container, blend all wet components.
2. In another container, blend all dry components.
3. Blend wet and dry components.
4. Fold in blueberries and mix well.
5. Pour mixture into 8-12 prepared muffin cups, fill 2/3 of the cups.
6. Bake for eighteen-twenty mins at 375 deg.F, when ready take out, and serve.

Nutrition: Calories 130; Fat 12 gm; Carbohydrates 0 gm; Protein 1 gm

238. Raisin Muffin

Preparation Time: ten mins

Cooking Time: twenty mins

Servings: eight-twelve

Ingredients:

- 2 eggs
- one tbsp olive oil
- one teacup milk
- two teacups whole wheat flour
- one tsp baking soda
- quarter tsp baking soda
- one tsp cinnamon
- one teacup raisins

Directions:

1. In a container, blend all wet components.
2. In another container, blend all dry components.
3. Blend wet and dry components.
4. Fold in blueberries and mix well.
5. Pour mixture into 8-12 prepared muffin cups, fill 2/3 of the cups.
6. Bake for eighteen-twenty mins at 375 deg.F, when ready take out, and serve.

Nutrition: Calories 502; Fat 17 gm; Carbohydrates 79 gm; Protein 3.9 gm

239. Parmesan Omelet

Preparation Time: five mins

Cooking Time: ten mins

Servings: one

Ingredients:

- 2 eggs
- quarter tsp salt
- quarter tsp black pepper
- one tbsp olive oil
- quarter teacup parmesan cheese
- quarter tsp basil

Directions:

1. In a container, blend all components and mix well.
2. In a griddle, heat olive oil and pour the egg mixture.
3. Cook for one-two mins on all sides.
4. When ready, take out the omelet from the griddle and serve.

Nutrition: Calories 291; Fat 21.7 gm; Carbohydrates 1.9 gm; Protein 22 gm

240. Asparagus Omelet

Preparation Time: five mins

Cooking Time: ten mins

Servings: one

Ingredients:

- 2 eggs
- quarter tsp salt
- quarter tsp black pepper
- one tbsp olive oil
- quarter teacup cheese
- quarter tsp basil
- one teacup asparagus

Directions:

1. In a container, blend all components and mix well.
2. In a griddle, heat olive oil and pour the egg mixture.
3. Cook for one-two mins on all sides.
4. When ready, take out the omelet from the griddle and serve.

Nutrition: Calories 102.5; Fat 5.1 gm; Carbohydrates 3.3 gm; Protein 10.3 gm

241. Onion Omelet

Preparation Time: five mins

Cooking Time: ten mins

Servings: one

Ingredients:

- 2 eggs
- quarter tsp salt
- quarter tsp black pepper
- one tbsp olive oil
- quarter teacup cheese
- quarter tsp basil
- one teacup red onion

Directions:

1. In a container, blend all components and mix well.
2. In a griddle, heat olive oil and pour the egg mixture.
3. Cook for one-two mins on all sides.
4. When ready, take out the omelet from the griddle and serve.

Nutrition: Calories 200; Fat 15 gm; Carbohydrates 4.6 gm; Protein 7.2 gm

242. Olive Omelet

Preparation Time: five mins

Cooking Time: ten mins

Servings: one

Ingredients:

- 2 eggs
- quarter tsp salt
- quarter tsp black pepper
- one tbsp olive oil
- quarter teacup cheese
- quarter tsp basil
- half teacup olives

Directions:

1. In a container, blend all components and mix well.
2. In a griddle, heat olive oil and pour the egg mixture.
3. Cook for one-two mins on all sides.
4. When ready, take out the omelet from the griddle and serve.

Nutrition: Calories 183; Fat 13.8 gm; Carbohydrates 4 gm; Protein 15 gm

243. Tomato Omelet

Preparation Time: five mins

Cooking Time: ten mins

Servings: one

Ingredients:

- 2 eggs
- quarter tsp salt
- quarter tsp black pepper
- one tbsp olive oil
- quarter teacup cheese
- quarter tsp basil
- one teacup tomatoes

Directions:

1. In a container, blend all components and mix well.
2. In a griddle, heat olive oil and pour the egg mixture.
3. Cook for one-two mins on all sides.
4. When ready, take out the omelet from the griddle and serve.

Nutrition: Calories 456; Fat 33 gm; Carbohydrates 13 gm; Protein 18.4 gm

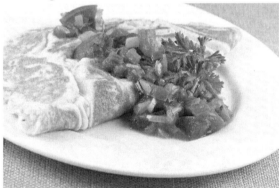

244. Morning Bagel

Preparation Time: five mins

Cooking Time: five mins

Servings: one

Ingredients:

- 1 bagel
- one tbsp cream cheese
- 2-3 tomato slices
- 1-2 onion slices

Directions:

1. Slice bagel and spread cream cheese over half.
2. Place tomato slices and onion over one half.
3. Top with the other half and serve.

Nutrition: Calories 289; Fat 2 gm; Carbohydrates 56 gm; Protein 11 gm

245. Oatmeal Custard

Preparation Time: five mins

Cooking Time: five mins

Servings: one

Ingredients:

- half teacup oatmeal
- quarter teacup coconut milk
- quarter tsp cinnamon
- ¼ pear

Directions:

1. In a mug, blend oats, milk, pear, and almonds.
2. Microwave for three to four mins.
3. When ready, take out and serve.

Nutrition: Calories 140; Fat 2.5 gm; Carbohydrates 28 gm; Protein 5 gm

246. Scrambled Eggs

Preparation Time: ten mins

Cooking Time: ten mins

Servings: one

Ingredients:

- 6 eggs
- half teacup low-fat milk
- quarter tsp salt
- quarter tsp pepper
- one tbsp butter
- half teacup cream cheese
- half teacup parmesan cheese

Directions:

1. In a container, whisk together eggs, salt, milk, and pepper.
2. In a griddle, pour the egg mixture and sprinkle cream cheese and cook for two-three mins on all sides.
3. Take out and serve with parmesan cheese.

Nutrition: Calories 91; Fat 6.7 gm; Carbohydrates 1.6 gm; Protein 10 gm

247. French Toast

Preparation Time: five mins

Cooking Time: ten mins

Servings: two

Ingredients:

- 2 bread slices
- one tsp unsalted butter

- 1 egg
- ½ almond milk

Directions:

1. In a container, blend all components for the dipping.
2. Place the bread slices in the container and let the bread soak for three to four mins.
3. Fry in a griddle for two-three mins on all sides.
4. When ready, take out from the griddle and serve.

Nutrition: Calories 229; Fat 11 gm; Carbohydrates 25 gm; Protein 8 gm

248. Simple Pizza Recipe

Preparation Time: 10mins

Cooking Time: fifteen mins

Servings: six-eight

Ingredients:

- 1 pizza crust
- half teacup tomato sauce
- ¼ black pepper
- one teacup pepperoni slices
- one teacup Mozzarella cheese
- one teacup olives

Directions:

1. Spread tomato sauce on the pizza crust.
2. Put the entire the toppings on the pizza crust.
3. Bake the pizza at 425 deg.F, for twelve-fifteen mins.
4. When ready, take out pizza from the oven and serve.

Nutrition: Calories 266; Fat 10 gm; Carbohydrates 33 gm; Protein 11 gm

249. Zucchini Pizza

Preparation Time: ten mins

Cooking Time: fifteen mins

Servings: six-eight

Ingredients:

- 1 pizza crust
- half teacup tomato sauce
- ¼ black pepper
- one teacup zucchini slices
- one teacup mozzarella cheese
- one teacup olives

Directions:

1. Spread tomato sauce on the pizza crust
2. Put the entire the toppings on the pizza crust
3. Bake the pizza at 425 deg.F for twelve-fifteen mins.
4. When ready, take out pizza from the oven and serve

Nutrition:

Calories 121; Fat 13 gm; Carbohydrates 31 gm; Protein 11 gm

250. Leeks Frittata

Preparation Time: ten mins

Cooking Time: twenty mins

Servings: two

Ingredients:

- half lbs. leek
- one tbsp olive oil
- ½ red onion
- quarter tsp salt
- 2 eggs
- 2 oz. Cheddar cheese
- 1 garlic piece
- quarter tsp dill

Directions:

1. In a container, whisk eggs with salt and cheese
2. In a frying pan, heat olive oil and pour egg mixture
3. Include rest of the components and mix well
4. Serve when ready

Nutrition: Calories 225; Fat 14.3 gm; Carbohydrates 9.7 gm; Protein 15 gm

251. Mushroom Fritatta

Preparation Time: ten mins

Cooking Time: twenty mins

Servings: two

Ingredients:

- half lbs. mushrooms
- one tbsp olive oil
- ½ red onion
- quarter tsp salt
- 2 eggs
- 2 oz. Cheddar cheese
- 1 garlic piece
- quarter tsp dill

Directions:

1. In a container, whisk eggs with salt and cheese
2. In a frying pan, heat olive oil and pour egg mixture
3. Include rest of the components and mix well
4. Serve when ready

Nutrition: Calories: 456; Carbohydrates: 26gm; Fats: 12gm; Protein: 7gm

252. Peas Frittata

Preparation Time: ten mins

Cooking Time: twenty mins

Servings: two

Ingredients:

- one teacup peas
- one tbsp olive oil
- ½ red onion
- quarter tsp salt

- 2 eggs
- 2 oz. Cheddar cheese
- 1 garlic piece
- quarter tsp dill

Directions:

1. In a container, whisk eggs with salt and cheese
2. In a frying pan, heat olive oil and pour egg mixture
3. Include rest of the components and mix well
4. Serve when ready

Nutrition:

Calories: 110; Fat: 6.2 gm; Carbohydrates: 4.9 gm; Protein: 8.5 gm

Lunch

253. High-Fiber Dumplings

Preparation Time: ten mins

Cooking Time: ten mins

Servings: eight

Ingredients:

- 200 gm cream quark
- 60 gm psyllium husks
- 10 gm bamboo fibers
- 1 container vegetable broth
- 2 eggs

Directions:

1. Take a container and include the psyllium husks along with the bamboo fibers. Mix well with a spoon.
2. Put the eggs in the same container, include the cream curd and vegetable stock. Knead well, its best done by hand. Alternatively, the kneading hooks of the mixer can be used.
3. Set a big saucepan with water and bring to a boil on the stove. In the meantime, moisten your hands with water and roll the dough into 12 balls.
4. Put the balls in the hot water and cook for ten mins, then serve. High-fiber vegetables like beans and matching sauces also taste great.

Nutrition: Calories: 75; Carbs: 0.1 gm; Protein: 13.4 gm; Fat: 1.7 gm; Sugar: 0 gm; Sodium: 253 mg

254. Pizza Made with Bamboo Fibers

Preparation Time: ten mins

Cooking Time: twenty mins

Servings: four

Ingredients:

- 2 eggs
- 60 gm bamboo fibers
- 80 gm sour cream
- 40 gm olive oil
- 150 gm grated Gouda cheese
- Salt and pepper

Directions:

1. First, preheat the oven to 180°C and cover a baking sheet with baking paper.

2. Take a container and beat in the eggs. Whisk briefly with a fork, then include the rest of the components and knead everything well. This is best done by hand, but you can also work with the dough hook on the mixer.

3. Finally, flavor with salt and pepper as required, then place the dough on the baking tray and roll out evenly. If necessary, flour the dough with a little bamboo fiber so that the dough does not stick to the rolling pin.

4. Bake the tray for ten mins on the lower rack. The pizza base can now be topped with delicious low-carb foods, depending on your taste. Then bake for an extra ten mins on the lower rack and then relish hot.

Nutrition: Calories: 599; Fat: 19 gm; Carbs: 9 gm; Sugar: 4 gm; Fiber: 2 gm; Protein: 97 gm; Sodium: 520 mg

255. **Vegetarian Hamburgers**

Preparation Time: ten mins

Cooking Time: thirty mins

Servings: four

Ingredients:

- 90 gm protein flour
- 120 ml egg white
- 100 gm carrots, grated
- two tbsps coconut oil
- 100 gm low-fat quark
- 2 eggs
- 6 gm baking powder
- 20 gm gold linseed (alternatively other nuts and grains)
- Preferred spices (Worcester sauce, soy sauce, salt, or chili)
- Preferred topping (tomatoes, cucumbers, radishes, ...)

Directions:

1. First, preheat the oven to 180°C and line 6-7 muffin tins with paper cases.

2. Take a container, include 50 gm of flour along with the egg white and carrots, and then stir well. Divide the dough into 6-7 parts and shape a meatball from each one.

3. Now, put two tbsps of coconut oil in a non-stick pan and heat at middling temp. till it has melted. Put the meatballs in the hot pan and fry vigorously on both sides.

4. Take a separate container, include the rest of the flour along with the low-fat quark, eggs, baking powder, and gold linseed.

5. Mix well, then pour into the prepared muffin cups. Bake in the oven for twenty-five mins, let the finished

rolls cool down well. Finally, cut the rolls in half with a sharp knife, top with a meatball of your choice, and season. Then, skewer the finished burger with a toothpick and relish.

Nutrition: Calories: 178; Fat: 4 gm; Carbs: 7 gm; Fiber: 2 gm; Protein: 27 gm

256. **Pork Steaks with Avocado**

Preparation Time: ten mins

Cooking Time: thirty mins

Servings: eight

Ingredients:

For the salsa:

- 6 limes
- three tbsps fruity olive oil
- 1 ½ dried chili pepper
- Salt and freshly ground pepper
- 2 mangoes (ripe, but still firm)
- 2 shallots
- 2 avocados
- A bunch coriander

For the steaks:

- 4 pork neck steaks (approximately 150 gm each)
- one tsp ground anise
- one tsp ground cumin
- Salt
- Freshly ground pepper
- two tbsps clarified butter

Directions:

For the salsa:

1. Halve the limes and squeeze them thoroughly, measure out 10 tablespoons of lime juice. Place in a small container.

2. Include olive oil and stir well with a whisker. Crumble the chili pepper and mix it into the dressing together with salt and pepper.

3. Now, peel the mangoes with a vegetable peeler, take out the stone and dice the pulp. Finely chop the shallots with a sharp knife.

4. Take a separate container, include the mangoes and shallots: stir well.

5. Take out the stone and skin from the avocados, dice the meat and then fill the mango mixture. Immediately, pour the dressing over it so that the avocado doesn't tarnish. Mix gently.

6. Finally, wash the coriander thoroughly under running water and dry it carefully. Take out the tender leaves and also include to the salsa. Mix again.

For the steaks:

1. Warm up the oven to 60°C. Rinse the steaks under running water and dry them carefully with a little kitchen roll. Spray the anise, cumin, salt, and pepper

over them. Place the clarified butter in a pan and heat at middling temp. till melted. Set the steaks in the hot pan and fry briefly while turning for three mins.

2. Put the steaks on a piece of aluminum foil and seal it tightly around the steak. Place in the oven and let rest briefly for three mins.

3. Arrange on a plate with the meat juice and salsa. Relish immediately!

Nutrition: Calories: 303; Fat: 14 gm; Carbs: 15 gm; Sugar: 10 gm; Fiber: 2 gm; Protein: 30 gm; Sodium: 387 mg

257. <u>Chicken with Asparagus Salad</u>

Preparation Time: ten mins

Cooking Time: thirty mins

Servings: four

Ingredients:

- 800 gm green asparagus
- 1/2 bunch spring onions
- three tbsps white wine vinegar
- Salt
- Pepper
- one tsp mustard
- half tsp honey
- eight tbsps olive oil
- 4 chicken breast fillets (approximately 200 gm each)
- 250 gm sliced breakfast bacon
- two tbsps clarified butter
- Basil leaves for garnishing

Directions:

1. First, preheat the oven to 180ºC and place baking paper on a baking sheet.

2. Take the asparagus and peel only the bottom stick.

3. Take out the woody ends, then wash thoroughly. Halve the asparagus lengthways and cut so that oblique pieces are created. Now, wash the spring onions and cut them into big pieces.

4. Take a container, pour the white wine vinegar into it. Also, attach two tbsps of water along with mustard, honey, salt, and pepper. Stir well.

5. Finally, slowly include 6 tablespoons of olive oil, spoon by spoon. Stir.

6. Take the meat, rinse under running water and dry with a little kitchen roll, then season with salt and pepper on both sides.

7. Take the bacon slices and wrap the meat in them.

8. Put the clarified butter in a non-stick pan and heat over medium fire till the fat has melted. Set the chicken breasts in the hot pan, first placing them to the point where the ends of the bacon slice meet. Turn after two mins and fry again briefly for two mins.

9. Take out from the pan and place on the tray so that the meat can cook in the oven for an extra fifteen mins.

10. In the meantime, set the rest of the olive oil in a pan and heat over medium fire. Put the vegetables in the hot oil and fry briefly. Meanwhile, salt and pepper. After 4 mins, take the vegetables out of the pan and include them to the vinegar mixture, mix well.

11. Finally, arrange the meat with the asparagus salad on a plate and relish immediately.

Nutrition:

Calories: 276; Fat: 15 gm; Carbs: 19 gm; Sugar: 10 gm; Fiber: 5 gm; Protein: 32 gm

258. <u>Hot Pepper and Lamb Salmon</u>

Preparation Time: ten mins

Cooking Time: twenty mins

Servings: six

Ingredients:

For the meat:

- 700 gm lamb salmon
- 2 garlic pieces
- 1/2 bunch mint
- 2 rosemary springs
- 1/2 bunch oregano
- 10 peppercorns
- 4 tablespoons olive oil
- Salt
- Pepper

For the Peperonata:

- 1 small zucchini
- 2 red peppers
- 2 yellow peppers
- 1 onion
- 3 garlic pieces
- 3 tomatoes
- 1 chili pepper
- three tbsps small capers
- two tbsps olive oil
- Salt
- Pepper
- two tbsps severed parsley

Directions:

For the meat:

1. First, rinse the meat under running water and dry it with a little kitchen roll, then carefully take out the tendons and fat. Peel and cut the garlic to make fine slices.

2. Wash the rosemary, oregano, and mint, pat dry carefully. Then, chop the leaves and needles (not too

fine). Put the peppercorns in the mortar and press lightly. Take a container, include the herbs and peppercorns.

3. Include two tbsps of olive oil and stir well, then rub the meat with the mixture. Finally, wrap it in foil and put in the fridge for four hrs.

4. Warm up the oven to 70 deg.C, placing a baking dish in it that will be used for the meat later.

5. Now, take the meat and take out the marinade with the back of a knife, then season with salt and pepper. Set the rest of the oil in a pan and heat over medium fire.

6. Place the meat in the hot oil and fry briefly while turning for two mins. Put it in the pan into the oven and cook for an extra forty mins.

For the Peperonata:

1. Wash the zucchini thoroughly and dice it with the skin. Halve and core the peppers, wash them too. Cut so that narrow strips are created. First, peel the onion and garlic then process into fine cubes.

2. Score the tomatoes, pour hot water, at that time peel them and take out the seeds. Cut the pulp into small pieces. Alternatively, canned tomatoes can also be used here. Halve and core the chili pepper, wash it well, and cut it into small pieces. Finally, rinse the capers in a sieve and let them drain.

3. Now, pour olive oil over the pan and heat over medium fire. Put the onion in the hot oil and fry briefly, then include the peppers, zucchini, garlic, and chili. Cook for five mins, stirring evenly. Attach tomatoes and season with salt and pepper.

4. Let everything fry for ten mins, stir in the capers and cook for an extra five mins.

Nutrition: Calories: 599; Fat: 19 gm; Carbs: 9 gm; Sugar: 4 gm; Fiber: 2 gm; Protein: 97 gm; Sodium: 520 mg

259. Pork Rolls à la Ratatouille

Preparation Time: ten mins

Cooking Time: thirty mins

Servings: eight

Ingredients:

For the Ratatouille:

- 2 yellow peppers
- 2 red peppers
- 2 small zucchini
- 2 red onions
- 3 garlic pieces
- 250 gm cherry tomatoes
- A bunch of thyme
- three tbsps olive oil
- Salt
- Freshly ground pepper
- 250 ml vegetable stock
- three tbsps tomato paste

For the Pork Rolls:

- 2 bunches basil
- 30 gm Parmesan cheese
- 30 gm pine nuts
- 5 tablespoons olive oil
- Salt
- Freshly ground pepper
- 75 gm sun-dried tomatoes in oil
- 8 small pork schnitzel (approximately 75 gm each)

Directions:

For the Ratatouille:

1. First, preheat the oven to 180ºC.

2. Halve and core the peppers, wash thoroughly, and cut so that narrow strips are formed.

3. Wash the zucchini as well, then cut into cubes with the skin on. First, peel the onion and garlic then cut into strips. Clean the tomatoes thoroughly, cut them in half.

4. Rinse the thyme under running water and pat dry carefully, take out the leaves. Take a container, include the vegetables with the thyme and mix well.

5. Flavor with salt, pepper, and olive oil. Mix again. Take the frying pan from the oven and distribute the vegetable mixture in it. Bake for twenty mins.

For the Pork Rolls:

1. Now, rinse the basil with water and shake dry, pluck the leaves and chop finely. Coarsely or finely grate the Parmesan with the grater as required.

2. Take a small pan, include the pine nuts and briefly toast them without adding any further fat, then put them in the blender. Also, include half of the severed basil along with the Parmesan and three tbsps of olive oil. Puree everything into a pesto, then season with salt and pepper.

3. Wash the tomatoes and cut them to make strips. Clean the pork as well, dry it with a little kitchen roll, and then plate with a meat tenderizer or a saucepan. Spray with salt and pepper, spread some pesto on top.

4. Spread the sun-dried tomatoes and the rest of the basil on top, roll into roulades and set. Include the rest of the oil to a pan and heat over medium fire, place the rolls in the hot oil and fry on all sides for five mins.

5. Take a small container, include the vegetable stock and tomato paste. Stir.

6. Include the cherry tomatoes and the mixture to the cooked vegetables in the oven. Put the meat on it and bake for an extra fifteen mins. Relish served on a plate with the rest of the pesto.

Nutrition: Calories: 280; Fat: 16 gm; Carbs: 5 gm; Sugar: 1 gm; Fiber: 0 gm; Protein: 29 gm

260. Pepper Fillet with Leek

Preparation Time: ten mins

Cooking Time: thirty mins

Servings: eight

Ingredients:

For the vegetables:

- 50 gm sun-dried tomatoes
- 100 gm pine nuts
- four big leeks
- two tbsps raisins
- two teacups peppercorns
- two tbsps olive oil
- Salt
- Freshly ground pepper

For the meat:

- two tbsps black pepper
- 4 tablespoons sesame seeds
- one tsp salt
- 4 sprigs rosemary
- 4 beef fillet steaks (approximately 180 gm each)
- 4 tablespoons sunflower oil

Directions:

1. Place the tomatoes in a heat-resistant container and pour boiling water over them. Let stand for ten mins, then take out the tomatoes and chop with a sharp knife.
2. Now, put the pine nuts in a small pan and briefly toast them without adding any further fat, stirring well. Set aside and wash the leek thoroughly and cut so that rings are formed. Rinse the raisins under cold running water.
3. Take a non-stick pan and pour in olive oil. Heat on high and include the leek. Saute briefly, include tomatoes and raisins at low temp. and stir well. Cook for ten mins, season with salt and pepper. Include the pine nuts then carefully stir in.
4. At the same time, put the peppercorns in the mortar and coarsely crush them, stirring in a small container with salt and sesame seeds.
5. Rinse off the rosemary and steaks then dry them with a little paper towel. Place the steaks with the edges in the pepper mixture so that the spices stick to the edges.
6. Now, heat oil in a non-stick pan on a high level and sear the meat on both sides for three mins. Immediately, wrap in a piece of aluminum foil, covering a sprig of rosemary with it.
7. After resting for five mins, take out the steaks and arrange them on a plate with the leek vegetables. Garnish with meat juice and relish instantly.

Nutrition: Calories: 504; Fat: 39 gm; Carbs: 10 gm; Sugar: 1 gm; Fiber: 2 gm; Protein: 28 gm; Sodium: 755 mg

261. Lamb Chops with Beans

Preparation Time: ten mins

Cooking Time: fifty mins

Servings: eight

Ingredients:

- 1 kg lamb chops
- 2 lemons juice
- Salt
- Pepper
- 150 ml olive oil (approximately)
- 6 garlic pieces
- 6 sprigs rosemary
- 6 sprigs thyme
- 2 onions
- 12 cocktail tomatoes
- 300 gm green beans
- 2 shallots
- 70 gm bacon
- two tsps butter
- Savory, as required

Directions:

1. First, rinse the lamb chops briefly under running water and carefully dry them with a little kitchen roll. Pour the lemon juice into a small container, include 100 ml of olive oil, salt, and pepper: stir well. Take the garlic and take out the peel. Cut so that thin slices are formed, also include to the lemon marinade.
2. Now, put the marinade together with the chops in a freezer bag, squeeze out the air, and seal.
3. Set aside for almost two hrs and let it soak in.
4. Warm up the oven to 180 deg.C. Rinse the rosemary, thyme, and pat dry. Take a baking dish and grease it with olive oil. Spread the herb sprigs in it.
5. Include the onions and cut into 4 parts, place them in the mold as well. Wash the tomatoes thoroughly and cut in half depending on the size, then include to the onions.
6. Set the meat out of the marinade and place it on top of the vegetables. Spread the soak and a little olive oil on top. Bake on the middle rack for forty mins.
7. In the meantime, take the beans and cut the ends, then wash. Set the water to a boil in a saucepan, season with salt, and include the beans. Cook for eight mins. Meanwhile, take the shallots and take out the skin, cut into small cubes. Finely dice the bacon as well.
8. Put the butter in a pan and heat over medium fire till it has melted.
9. Place the shallots and bacon in the hot oil and fry till everything takes on a brown color.
10. Include the beans with a little savory, stir well.

11. Salt and pepper, then serve with the lamb and the bed of vegetables. Relish hot.

Nutrition: Calories: 413; Fat: 20 gm; Carbs: 7 gm; Sugar: 1 gm; Fiber: 1 gm; Protein: 50 gm; Sodium: 358 mg

262. Fillet of Beef on Spring Vegetables

Preparation Time: ten mins

Cooking Time: thirty mins

Servings: eight

Ingredients:

- 500 gm green asparagus
- 2 bulbs kohlrabi
- 1 bunch flat-leaf parsley
- 1 bunch tarragon
- Salt
- Pepper
- 4 beef fillet steaks (approximately 150 gm each)
- 4 tablespoons olive oil
- 300 ml cream

Directions:

1. Wash the asparagus, peel only the bottom stick, with the vegetable peeler. Divide off the woody ends, then cut the asparagus in half. Now, peel the kohlrabi with the knife, cut so that narrow sticks are formed.
2. Rinse the herbs under running water, dry them carefully and take out the leaves. Finely chop with a sharp knife. Take a container, pour in 2/3 of the herbs, put away the rest for now.
3. After that, include the vegetables to the herbs in the container, season with salt and pepper, and mix well. Put the mixture in a roasting tube (must be closed on one side).
4. Take a big saucepan, pour water up to 1/3 full. Set on the stove and bring to a boil.
5. In the meantime, rinse the steaks with water and dry them carefully with a little kitchen roll.
6. Season with salt and pepper on both sides. Put the oil in a pan and heat over medium fire.
7. Set the meat in the hot oil and fry briefly on all sides for three mins. Place it on the vegetables in the roasting tube.
8. Pour the oil out of the pan and include in the cream. Bring to the boil briefly so that the roasting loosens, then pour over the meat in the roasting tube.
9. Now, close the hose and include it to the boiling water. Cook gently at low temp. and cover for 1two mins.
10. Finally, arrange the meat with the bed of vegetables on a plate and garnish with the rest of the herbs.

Nutrition: Calories: 209; Fat: 10 gm; Carbs: 21 gm; Sugar: 13 gm; Fiber: 8 gm; Protein: 11 gm; Sodium: 644 mg

263. Bolognese with Zucchini Noodles

Preparation Time: ten mins

Cooking Time: fifty mins

Servings: four-eight

Ingredients:

- 4 zucchinis (approximately 200 gm each)
- Salt
- 1 onion
- 3 garlic pieces
- two tbsps coconut oil
- 4 tablespoons tomato paste
- three tbsps balsamic vinegar
- 600 gm chunky tomatoes, canned
- 4 sprigs rosemary
- 1 handful basil leaves
- ½ tablespoon dried oregano
- quarter tsp dried thyme
- Freshly ground black pepper
- 600 gm mixed crushed meat
- two tbsps olive oil

Directions:

1. First, wash the zucchini and cut them into thin, narrow slices.
2. For preparing the Bolognese, peel the onion and garlic: cut into fine cubes. Set the oil in a saucepan and heat over medium fire. Put the onion in the hot oil and fry till it becomes translucent.
3. Stir well and fry briefly prior to adding the tomato paste. Cook them together again, pour in the balsamic vinegar till the bottom can no longer be seen. Bring to a boil, include the tomatoes.
4. Wash the rosemary, and basil then dry them carefully. Pluck the needles and leaves, chop and include to the Bolognese. Season with the rest of the herbs as required.
5. Reduce the heat and simmer gently for thirty mins prior to stirring in the crushed meat. Cook for an extra fifteen mins, then cook at high heat for five mins.
6. At the same time, attach olive oil to the zucchini noodles and mix well.
7. Put the oiled zucchini in a pan and cook only briefly at middling temp. without becoming too soft.
8. Arrange with the Bolognese on a plate. Relish hot.

Nutrition: Calories: 75; Carbs: 0.1 gm; Protein: 13.4 gm; Fat: 1.7 gm; Sugar: 0 gm; Sodium: 253 mg

264. Chicken with Chickpeas

Preparation Time: ten mins

Cooking Time: thirty mins

Servings: four

Ingredients:

- 12 sun-dried tomatoes in oil
- 2 garlic pieces

- 2 zucchini
- 500 gm chickpeas (canned, drained weight)
- 4 tablespoons olive oil
- 100 ml poultry stock
- 2 bags saffron threads
- Salt
- Freshly ground black pepper
- quarter tsp ground coriander
- 4 chicken breasts (approximately 200 gm each)
- one tbsp Ras el Hanout

Directions:

1. First, get the sun-dried tomatoes out of the oil and dry them with a little kitchen roll, then cut them so that narrow strips are formed.
2. Take the garlic, take out the skin and cut it into slices.
3. Wash the zucchini and cut into cubes with the skin on.
4. Rinse the chickpeas in a colander and drain well.
5. Set a saucepan, include two tbsps of olive oil. Warmth on medium heat, include the tomatoes with garlic to the hot oil. Fry briefly for one min.
6. Place the zucchini with chickpeas, stir well and fry briefly together prior to deglazing with the broth. Include saffron threads, coriander, salt, and pepper. Bring to a boil.
7. Set the heat, cover the saucepan and let the vegetables simmer for five mins.
8. In the meantime, rinse the meat under running water and dry it with a little kitchen roll. Set the rest of the oil in a pan and heat over medium fire.
9. For now, sprinkle the meat on both sides with salt, pepper, and Ras el Hanout. Then, include to the hot oil and fry for seven mins, turning.
10. Serve the meat with the vegetables on a big plate. Relish hot.

Nutrition: Calories: 329; Fat: 17 gm; Carbs: 9 gm; Sugar: 3 gm; Fiber: 5 gm; Protein: 37 gm; Sodium: 430 mg

265. Ham with Chicory

Preparation Time: ten mins

Cooking Time: thirty mins

Servings: four-eight

Ingredients:

- 4 chicory sprigs (approximately 200 gm each)
- 150 gm Emmental cheese
- 8 sage leaves
- 40 gm butter
- three tbsps orange juice
- Salt
- Pepper
- 8 slices Black Forest ham

Directions:

1. First, preheat the oven to 200ºC.
2. Wash and clean the chicory and cut it lengthways in half. Take out the stalk with a knife.
3. Shred the cheese coarsely or finely with a grater as required.
4. Rinse the sage leaves under running water and gently shake dry.
5. Put the butter in a pan and heat over medium fire. Extinguish with orange juice and froth the butter. Include the sage.
6. Place the chicory with the cut side in the hot oil. Reduce the heat and fry for five mins.
7. Take out the chicory, cover with a sage leaf and sprinkle with salt and pepper.
8. Chop the ham and put it on the baking dish. Spray with cheese and drizzle with liquid orange and butter. Bake in the oven for twenty mins, then serve hot.

Nutrition: Calories: 75; Carbs: 0.1 gm; Protein: 13.4 gm; Fat: 1.7 gm; Sugar: 0 gm; Sodium: 253 mg

266. Pork Medallions with Asparagus and Coconut Curry

Preparation Time: ten mins

Cooking Time: thirty mins

Servings: four-eight

Ingredients:

- 1 kg white asparagus
- 500 gm carrots
- 2 onions
- 1 red chili pepper
- 40 gm butter
- three to four tablespoons curry powder
- 250 ml vegetable stock
- 400 ml coconut milk
- two–three tbsps lime juice
- Salt
- Pepper
- one tbsp severed coriander
- 4 pork medallions (125 gm each)
- two-three tbsps oil

Directions:

1. First, peel the asparagus and take out the woody ends, wash well and cut into bite-sized pieces. Then, peel the carrots, wash and cut them into slices. Now, take the onions, take out the skin, and cut them into cubes. Divide the chili in half, take out the seeds, and carefully dice.
2. Put the butter in a pan. Heat over medium fire till it has melted.

3. Put the onions and chili in the hot oil and sauté till translucent. Include asparagus, carrots and fry everything for five mins, stirring regularly.

4. Pour the curry over it and fry briefly prior to adding the broth. Set the heat, cover the saucepan, and simmer for fifteen mins.

5. Include in the coconut milk and cook for additional three mins. Pour in lime juice, salt, and pepper as required. Spray on half tbsp of coriander. Stir well.

6. Now, take the meat and season with salt and pepper on both sides. Put the oil in a pan and heat over medium fire.

7. Place the medallions in the hot oil and fry briefly on both sides for around three-five mins.

8. Arrange medallions with curry on a plate. Garnish with coriander. Serve warm.

Nutrition: Calories: 432; Fat: 12 gm; Carbs: 12 gm; Sugar: 5 gm; Fiber: 3 gm; Protein: 57 gm; Sodium: 566 mg

267. Lamb with Carrot and Brussels Sprouts Spaghetti

Preparation Time: ten mins

Cooking Time: thirty mins

Servings: four-eight

Ingredients:

- 250 gm Brussels sprouts
- 300 gm carrots
- 5 tablespoons sesame oil
- three tbsps soy sauce
- 1 lime juice
- A tweak sugar
- Salt
- 600 gm loosened saddle lamb
- Pepper
- two tbsps butter
- two tbsps sesame seeds

Directions:

1. First, preheat the oven to 100°C.
2. Take the Brussels sprouts, wash, and clean. Then, cut them into strips.
3. For preparing the marinade, place three tbsps of sesame oil together with soy sauce, sugar, salt, and lime juice inside a container. Merge well.
4. Put the vegetable spaghetti in the marinade and let it steep for a moment.
5. In the meantime, flavor the lamb with salt and pepper. Pour the rest of the oil into a coated pan and heat on high.
6. Set the meat in the hot oil and sear it on all sides, then put it in the oven and let it cook gently for ten mins.
7. After that, melt the butter in the same pan and fry the marinated vegetables for around three to four mins.

Arrange on a plate with the sliced lamb and garnish with sesame seeds.

Nutrition: Calories: 270; Fat: 11 gm; Carbs: 4 gm; Sugar: 1 gm; Fiber: 1 gm; Protein: 39 gm; Sodium: 664 mg

268. Cabbage Wrap

Preparation Time: ten mins

Cooking Time: thirty mins

Servings: four-eight

Ingredients:

- 1 head white cabbage
- Salt
- 100 ml milk
- 1 roll (from the day prior to)
- 350 gm mixed crushed meat
- 1 egg freshly ground pepper
- two tbsps clarified butter
- 250 ml meat stock
- one tbsp flour
- 4 tablespoons cream

Directions:

1. First, separate the big outer leaves (12-16 pieces) from the cabbage and cut out the strong leaf veins with a knife. Set a saucepan with water and bring to a boil. Salt well and include the big cabbage leaves with the rest of the cabbage. Cook everything for five-ten mins.

2. Heat the milk in a saucepan. Put the roll on it and soak for a couple of mins.

3. Squeeze out the bun and place it inside a container. Also include the crushed meat, egg, pepper, and salt. Mix everything well till a batter is formed.

4. Cut the cooked cabbage (not the big leaves) and include to the dough, mix again.

5. Take three to four cabbage leaves and stack them on top of each other. Spread some batter on top, then roll the leaves and fix with toothpicks, roulade needles, or kitchen twine.

6. Put the clarified butter in a pan and heat over medium fire till it melts. Then, place the cabbage rolls in the hot oil and fry them lightly brown.

7. Extinguish with the broth, cover the pan, and simmer the cabbage rolls at low temp. for twenty-five mins. Take out the cabbage rolls and briefly keep them warm.

8. Now, stir in the flour in a little cream and include everything to the sauce. Bring to a boil briefly.

9. Arrange on plates with the cabbage rolls.

Nutrition: Calories: 329; Fat: 17 gm; Carbs: 9 gm; Sugar: 3 gm; Fiber: 5 gm; Protein: 37 gm

269. Veal with Asparagus

Preparation Time: ten mins

Cooking Time: thirty mins

Servings: four-eight

Ingredients:

- 800 gm green asparagus
- Salt
- three to four tablespoons rapeseed oil
- A tweak sugar
- Pepper
- 1/2 fresh lemon zest, grated
- Oil for frying
- 8 slices veal from the back (60 gm each)
- 8 slices Parma ham
- 8 sage leaves
- 125 ml white wine
- one tbsp butter

Directions:

1. First, peel the lower part of the sticks with a vegetable peeler, then take out the woody ends. Wash the asparagus thoroughly.
2. At the same time, fill a saucepan with water and bring it to a boil. Salt well, include the asparagus, and cook for eight mins. They must not become too soft. Drain them and rinse directly with ice water.
3. Place the asparagus on a piece of kitchen roll to dry, then put them in a baking dish.
4. Take a small container and include the oil, salt, pepper, sugar 0and lemon zest. Mix everything well and pour over the asparagus stalks. Let sit in the marinade for twenty-five mins.
5. Put the oil in a pan and heat over medium fire. Detach the asparagus from the marinade and place them in the hot oil. Fry while turning.
6. Now, pepper the meat and cover it with Parma ham and a sage leaf. Secure everything with a toothpick.
7. Put the oil in a pan, heat it and place the meat in it. Fry briefly on medium heat and turn for three mins.
8. Serve with the asparagus on a plate. Extinguish the now-empty pan with white wine so that the roasting residue dissolves, then stir in the butter and briefly bring to a boil.
9. Pour the sauce over the asparagus and meat. Relish hot.

Nutrition: Calories: 599; Fat: 19 gm; Carbs: 9 gm; Sugar: 4 gm; Fiber: 2 gm; Protein: 97 gm; Sodium: 520 mg

270. Salmon with Sesame Seeds and Mushrooms

Preparation Time: ten mins

Cooking Time: thirty mins

Servings: four-eight

Ingredients:

- 500 gm salmon fillet
- 4 tablespoons fish sauce
- 200 gm mushrooms
- 400 gm fresh spinach leaves
- two tbsps vegetable oil
- two tbsps sesame oil
- one tbsp sesame seeds
- one tsp sambal oelek

Directions:

1. First, take the salmon, rinse under running water, dry with a little kitchen roll, and then cut so that strips are formed. Take a container, pour in the fish sauce. Soak the salmon in the sauce for ten mins.
2. In the meantime, it is best to carefully clean the mushrooms with a brush, cut them to make slices. Rinse and dry the spinach under the tap.
3. Now, take a wok, include the vegetable and sesame oil. Heat on high, include the mushrooms to the hot oil and fry briefly. Put the spinach in the wok. Fry till it collapses.
4. Now, move the vegetables away from the center to the edge of the wok; reduce the heat.
5. Place the salmon on the resulting surface. Fry gently while turning.
6. Arrange it with the vegetables on a plate, and carefully refine with sambal oelek as required.

Nutrition: Calories: 599; Fat: 19 gm; Carbs: 9 gm; Sugar: 4 gm; Fiber: 2 gm; Protein: 97 gm; Sodium: 520 mg

271. Stuffed Trout with Mushrooms

Preparation Time: ten mins

Cooking Time: thirty mins

Servings: four-eight

Ingredients:

- 4 ready-to-cook trout
- 1 lemon juice
- Salt
- Pepper
- 1/2 bunch dill
- 500 gm mushrooms
- two tbsps butter
- two tbsps freshly severed parsley
- three tbsps severed almonds
- 4 tablespoons oil

Directions:

1. First, preheat the oven to 220°C.
2. Take the lemon juice and use it to drizzle the trout inside and out. Wash the dill, shake dry and chop.
3. Salt and pepper the trout and refine each with one tbsp of dill. It is best to carefully clean the mushrooms with a brush and cut them into slices.
4. Then, put them inside a container. Also include the butter, almonds, and parsley. Stir everything well.

5. Now, distribute the filling over the trout's abdominal cavities. Fix the abdomen with wooden skewers, wrap the trout well in aluminum foil coated with oil. Let it cook in the oven for twenty mins.

6. Finally, put the fish on a plate. Relish hot.

Nutrition: Calories: 413; Fat: 20 gm; Carbs: 7 gm; Sugar: 1 gm; Fiber: 1 gm; Protein: 50 gm; Sodium: 358 mg

272. **Salmon with Basil and Avocado**

Preparation Time: ten mins

Cooking Time: thirty mins

Servings: four-eight

Ingredients:

- 1 avocado
- one tsp pickled capers
- 3 garlic pieces
- A handful basil leaves
- one tbsp fresh lemon zest
- 4 salmon fillets (approximately 200 gm each)
- Coconut oil for greasing the tray

Directions:

1. Warm up the oven at 180°C. Use a brush to spread coconut oil on a baking sheet.
2. Divide the avocado in half, then take out the core and skin.
3. Mash the pulp with a fork in a small container.
4. Put the capers in a colander and drain, chop finely.
5. Peel the garlic pieces and mash them with a press. Alternatively, chop them very finely with a sharp knife.
6. Then, wash the basil and shake it dry, pluck the leaves off and chop them too.
7. Attach everything to the avocado in the container. Refine with lemon zest, and mix well.
8. Wash the salmon, dry with a little kitchen roll, and place on the baking sheet. It is best to spread the avocado mixture over the fish with a spoon.
9. Put the tray in the oven and bake briefly for ten mins. Switch on the grill function; bake for an extra four mins till the avocado takes on a light brown color.
10. Set the salmon fillets on a plate, and relish hot.

Nutrition: Calories: 209; Fat: 10 gm; Carbs: 21 gm; Sugar: 13 gm; Fiber: 8 gm; Protein: 11 gm; Sodium: 644 mg

273. **Leek Quiche with Olives**

Preparation Time: ten mins

Cooking Time: thirty mins

Servings: four-eight

Ingredients:

- 140 gm almonds
- 40 gm walnuts
- 25 gm coconut oil
- one tsp salt
- 1 leek
- 50 gm spinach
- 2 sprigs rosemary
- 40 gm fresh basil
- 30 gm pine nuts
- 4 tablespoons extra-virgin olive oil
- two tbsps lime juice
- 1/2 garlic piece
- 50 gm pitted black olives
- one tsp red pepper berries

Directions:

1. First, coarsely grind the almonds and walnuts inside a blending container or blender. Then, put them in a small container together with the coconut oil and half tsp of salt.
2. Merge thoroughly, pour the mixture into a cake spring-form pan. Press the dough with your fingers at the same time, and distribute it in the mold so that a border of 4 cm high is created. Put it in the freezer for fifteen mins.
3. Now, wash the leek, spinach, and herbs. Then, pat dry. Slice the leek and place it inside a container.
4. Stir in the rest of the salt and put away to draw.
5. Meanwhile, put the basil, pine nuts, olive oil, and lime juice in a blender. Pulse till you have a creamy puree.
6. Alternatively, a big mixing vessel or a hand blender can also be used here.
7. Now, peel the garlic piece and chop half. Take out the needles from the rosemary, and also finely chop them.
8. Cut the spinach into narrow strips and halve the olives.
9. Include everything to the leek in the container, and then include the basil puree. Mix well.
10. Distribute the mixture to the base of the spring-form pan. Spray with the pepper berries over it. Finally, cut the quiche into pieces and relish.

Nutrition: Calories: 270; Fat: 11 gm; Carbs: 4 gm; Sugar: 1 gm; Fiber: 1 gm; Protein: 39 gm; Sodium: 664 mg

274. **Fried Egg on Onions with Sage**

Preparation Time: ten mins

Cooking Time: thirty mins

Servings: four-eight

Ingredients:

- 275 gm onions
- 1/2 bunch sage
- three tbsps clarified butter
- 1 ½ tablespoon coconut flour
- Salt
- one tsp sweet paprika powder

- 8 eggs
- Freshly ground black pepper

Directions:

1. First, take out the skin from the onions; then, cut into thin rings.
2. Rinse the sage under running water, pat dry, and take out the leaves.
3. Now, put 1 ½ tablespoon of clarified butter in a pan. Heat over medium fire till it has melted. Place the sage leaves in the hot oil and fry till they are crispy. Place on kitchen paper to drain.
4. Meanwhile, put the rest of the clarified butter in the same pan and heat it. Then, place the onion rings in it.
5. Scatter the coconut flour on top and fry for ten mins, stirring at regular intervals. Spray salt and paprika too.
6. Take the eggs and beat them one by one on the onions in the pan. Let the eggs sink to the bottom of the pan, if necessary use a wooden spoon to help.
7. Now, cover the pan and fry everything for ten mins till the eggs are entirely set.
8. Arrange the fried eggs with the onions on flat plates. Season with salt and pepper. Garnish with the roasted sage.

Nutrition: Calories: 179; Fat: 13 gm; Carbs: 6 gm; Sugar: 3 gm; Fiber: 1 gm; Protein: 10 gm; Sodium: 265 mg

275. Quinoa Mushroom Risotto

Preparation Time: ten mins

Cooking Time: thirty mins

Servings: four-eight

Ingredients:

- 1 garlic piece
- 30 gm hazelnuts
- Salt
- 1 fresh lemon zest, grated
- 2 shallots
- 650 gm small mushrooms
- 1 bunch flat-leaf parsley
- 70 gm quinoa
- two tbsps olive oil
- Pepper
- 100 gm baby spinach
- 30 gm grated Parmesan cheese
- 20 gm butter
- Red pepper, as required
- 500 ml hot water

Directions:

1. First, peel the garlic piece and put it in a blender. Also include the hazelnuts, lemon zest, and a little salt. Mix till everything is finely ground. Put aside.

2. Peel the shallots, then cut them into fine cubes. It is best to carefully clean the mushrooms with a brush, chop them so that thin slices are formed.
3. Rinse and dab the parsley under running water. Take out the leaves and chop with a sharp knife.
4. Put the quinoa in a colander and wash well under the tap. Drain thoroughly.
5. Pour olive oil into a non-stick pan and warmth at middling temp.. Put the shallots in it, and fry till they turn slightly brown.
6. Include the mushrooms to the shallots and fry them together till they turn brown. Attach the quinoa, but at the same time pour in the hot water. Season with salt and pepper. Stir well.
7. Cook at low temp. till all the water has boiled away. The quinoa should be soft.
8. Now, include the parsley, spinach, Parmesan, and butter. Stir thoroughly.
9. Salt and pepper again. Set with garlic and the hazelnut mixture.
10. Arrange on a plate and serve garnished with red pepper, if necessary.

Nutrition: Calories: 166; Fat: 10 gm; Carbs: 17 gm; Sugar: 12 gm; Fiber: 2 gm; Protein: 7 gm; Sodium: 892 mg

276. Vegetarian Lentil Stew

Preparation Time: ten mins

Cooking Time: thirty mins

Servings: four

Ingredients:

- 50 gm carrots
- 30 gm parsnip or parsley root
- 30 gm celery
- 1 leek
- 1 yellow pepper
- 250 gm red lentils
- 1 half tsp ground cumin
- three tbsps balsamic vinegar
- three tbsps walnut oil
- two-three tbsps maple syrup
- Salt and pepper
- A tweak of cayenne pepper
- 1/2 bunch flat-leaf parsley

Directions:

1. Measure 1000 ml of water and pour into a saucepan. Warmth on high heat till boil.
2. In the meantime, cut the peppers in half, take out the seeds and wash them together with the leek. Peel the carrots, parsnips, and celery.
3. Process everything into fine cubes, only use the white part of the leek.

4. Pour everything into the boiling water and bring to a boil. Then, include the lentils. Cook for ten mins, or till they are soft.

5. Ideally, most of the liquid has boiled away, if necessary drain. Season with cumin, balsamic vinegar, maple syrup, walnut oil, salt, and pepper. Include the cayenne pepper as required.

6. Turn off the stove and set the vegetarian lentils stew aside briefly to steep.

7. In the meantime, rinse the parsley under the tap, pat dry, pluck the leaves off and sprinkle them into the stew.

8. Arrange in deep plates and relish hot.

Nutrition: Calories: 413; Fat: 20 gm; Carbs: 7 gm; Sugar: 1 gm; Fiber: 1 gm; Protein: 50 gm; Sodium: 358 mg

277. Lemon Chicken Soup with Beans

Preparation Time: ten mins

Cooking Time: fifty mins

Servings: four

Ingredients:

- 1 onion
- 6 garlic pieces
- 600 gm chicken breast
- three tbsps olive oil
- l chicken broth
- 1 fresh lemon
- 250 gm cooked white beans, canned
- Salt
- Pepper
- 120 gm Feta
- A bunch chive

Directions:

1. First, peel the onion, then the garlic pieces. Divide the onion in half and cut it into thin slices.

2. Rinse the meat under running water and dry it with a little paper towel.

3. Put the olive oil in a big saucepan and heat over medium fire. Include the onion and garlic to the hot oil.

4. Fry till everything is soft; deglaze with the chicken stock. Also, include the meat and bring it to a boil.

5. In the meantime, wash and dry the lemon, then rub and peel it with a grater, alternatively. You can also use a zester. Include the lemon zest to the broth and cook everything for forty mins prior to adding the beans. Salt and pepper, then cook again for ten mins.

6. Now, take out the meat and tear it into small pieces on a plate or board with 2 forks. Put the chicken back into the soup, then crumble the Feta over the soup.

7. Finally, rinse the chives with water. Dry and cut them so that small rolls are created. Spray into the soup; stir well and immediately relish hot.

Nutrition: Calories: 329; Fat: 17 gm; Carbs: 9 gm; Sugar: 3 gm; Fiber: 5 gm; Protein: 37 gm; Sodium: 430 mg

Snacks

278. Banana-Bread Muffins

Preparation Time: fifteen mins

Cooking Time: thirty mins

Servings: twelve

Ingredients:

- two teacups oat flour
- one tsp baking soda
- A tweak sea salt
- one tbsp ground cinnamon
- half teacup coconut oil
- 3 unripe bananas, mashed
- 2 eggs
- three-quarter teacup raw sugar
- quarter teacup maple syrup
- half tsp pure vanilla extract
- half teacup severed walnuts or pecans
- half teacup blueberries

Directions:

1. Warm up the oven to 325 deg.F. Line a muffin tin with paper liners.

2. Blend the oat flour, baking soda, salt, and cinnamon in a medium container. Set aside.

3. In a small microwave-safe container, melt the coconut oil in the microwave. Pour it into a big blending container. Include the mashed bananas, eggs, sugar, maple syrup, and vanilla. Mix well.

4. Include the dry components to the wet components. Stir till well blended. Gently fold in the walnuts and blueberries.

5. Fill each muffin cup three-quarters full. Bake for 25 to thirty mins, or till a toothpick inserted into the center of a muffin comes out clean.

Nutrition: Calories: 213; Carbohydrates: 29 gm; Fat: 11 gm; Protein: 2 gm; Fiber: 2 gm; Sodium: 135 mg

279. Berry Fruit Leathers

Preparation Time: five mins

Cooking Time: three hrs and thirty mins

Servings: six

Ingredients:

- two teacups strawberries
- two teacups blueberries
- half teacup maple syrup
- 1 lemon juice

Directions:

1. Warm up the oven to 200 deg.F. Line two baking sheets with parchment paper.

2. Include the strawberries, blueberries, maple syrup, and lemon juice to a blender, and blend till smooth.

3. Divide the mixture between the two small baking sheets and use a rubber spatula to spread it across the sheets in an even layer.

4. Bake for 3 to 3½ hours, or till no longer sticky when you tap it with your finger.

5. Let the berry leather cool for around thirty mins, then use a pizza cutter or scissors to cut it into 8 strips, each about one inch-wide and 5 inches long.

Nutrition: Calories: 38; Carbohydrates: 11 gm; Fat: 0 gm; Protein: 0.5 gm; Fiber: 1 gm; Sodium: 2 mg

280. Chocolate-Covered Banana Slices

Preparation Time: ten mins

Cooking Time: five mins

Servings: two

Ingredients:

- 1 unripe banana, frozen and sliced
- half teacup high-quality milk, or dark chocolate chips

Directions:

1. Line a baking sheet with parchment paper and place the banana slices on the sheet in a single layer separately.

2. In a microwave-safe container, melt the chocolate in the microwave at 30-second intervals, making sure to stir it between intervals.

3. Pour the chocolate over the banana slices till they're entirely covered.

4. Refrigerate for almost one hr till the chocolate hardens entirely. Transfer to a sealed container and put in the fridge for up to 1 week.

Nutrition: Calories: 333; Carbohydrates: 46 gm; Fat: 20 gm; Protein: 5 gm; Fiber: 6 gm; Sodium: 1 mg

281. Coconut Macaroons

Preparation Time: ten mins

Cooking Time: fifteen mins

Servings: twelve

Ingredients:

- 6 egg whites
- A tweak sea salt
- half teacup maple syrup
- one tbsp vanilla extract
- three teacups unsweetened shredded coconut

Directions:

1. Warm up the oven to 350 deg.F. Line two baking sheets with parchment paper.

2. In a small container, include the egg whites and salt. Using an electric mixer on high speed, whisk the eggs till firm peaks form, five to six mins.

3. Using a rubber spatula, gently fold in the maple syrup, vanilla, and coconut till well blended.

4. Drop 1 rounded tablespoon of batter at a time on the baking sheet, leaving about 2 inches between each macaroon.

5. Bake for twelve to fifteen mins, or till lightly browned.

Nutrition: Calories: 156; Carbohydrates: 13 gm; Fat: 10 gm; Protein: 3 gm; Fiber: 2 gm; Sodium: 42 mg

282. Banana Ice Cream

Preparation Time: five mins

Cooking Time: zero mins

Servings: two

Ingredients:

- 2 frozen bananas
- two tbsps cocoa powder
- two tbsps peanut butter
- one tsp maple syrup
- half tsp vanilla extract

Directions:

1. Put the frozen bananas, cocoa powder, peanut butter, maple syrup, and vanilla in a blender. Blend till smooth.

2. Serve immediately or freeze in a sealed, freezer-safe container.

Nutrition: Calories: 111; Carbohydrates: 18 gm; Fat: 5 gm; Protein: 3 gm; Fiber: 3 gm; Sodium: 38 mg

283. Berry-Berry Sorbet

Preparation Time: thirty mins

Cooking Time: zero mins

Servings: two

Ingredients:

- one teacup halved strawberries
- one teacup blueberries
- 1 lemon juice
- one-third teacup maple syrup

Directions:

1. Inside a mixer, include the strawberries, blueberries, lemon juice, and maple syrup. Blend till the mixture has a smooth and even texture.

2. Pour the mixture into an ice cream maker. Freeze the sorbet according to the manufacturer's instructions. It takes about twenty-five mins.

3. Transfer the sorbet into a sealed, freezer-safe container and let freeze for almost two hrs prior to serving.

Nutrition: Calories: 104; Carbohydrates: 26 gm; Fat: 0 gm; Protein: 1 gm; Fiber: 2 gm; Sodium: 5 mg

284. Oatmeal Semisweet Chocolate-Chip Cookies

Preparation Time: fifteen mins

Cooking Time: eleven mins

Servings: twelve

Ingredients:

- two and half teacups oat flour
- one tsp baking soda
- A tweak sea salt, plus extra for garnish
- half teacup coconut oil
- two-third teacup dark brown sugar
- 1 egg
- one tsp vanilla extract
- half teacup semisweet chocolate chips

Directions:

1. Warm up the oven to 350 deg.F. Line two baking sheets with parchment paper.
2. In a medium container, blend the oat flour, baking soda, and salt. Set aside.
3. In a microwave-safe container, melt the coconut oil; then, pour it into a big blending container.
4. To this big container, include the sugar, egg, and vanilla. Mix till well blended.
5. Include the dry components to the wet components. Mix well.
6. Fold in the chocolate chips till just blended.
7. Put tablespoon-size scoops of batter on the baking sheets, leaving about 2 inches between each cookie. Bake for around eleven mins, or till golden brown.
8. As soon as the cookies come out of the oven, sprinkle them with a little salt. Let the cookies cool on the pan for around two mins; then, transfer them to a wire rack to cool entirely.

Nutrition: Calories: 93; Carbohydrates: 9 gm; Fat: 6 gm; Protein: 1 gm; Fiber: 1 gm; Sodium: 67 mg

285. Coconut-Lemon Bars

Preparation Time: forty mins

Cooking Time: thirty-two mins

Servings: twelve

Ingredients:

For the crust

- Nonstick cooking spray
- one and half teacups old-fashioned oats
- half teacup unsweetened shredded coconut
- quarter teacup raw sugar
- A tweak sea salt
- quarter teacup coconut oil

For the filling

- 2 eggs
- half teacup raw sugar
- 5 tablespoons freshly squeezed lemon juice
- one tbsp freshly grated lemon zest
- one tsp vanilla extract
- two tbsps cornstarch

For the topping

- one-third teacup raw sugar
- quarter teacup freshly squeezed lemon juice
- quarter teacup water
- two tbsps cornstarch
- quarter teacup unsweetened shredded coconut

Directions:

To make the crust

1. Warm up the oven to 350 deg.F. Spray an 8-by-8-inch baking pan with the cooking spray.
2. Inside a blending container, include the oats, coconut, and sugar. Process till they're blended and ground to a fine texture.
3. In a microwave-safe container, melt the coconut oil in a microwave. Include the melted coconut oil to the food processor. Pulse till it's blended with the oat mixture.
4. Transfer the mixture to the baking pan and press it down with the back of a spoon till it covers the bottom of the pan in an even layer.
5. Bake for around fourteen mins, or till golden brown. Set aside to cool for almost twenty mins.

To make the filling

1. While the crust is cooling, include the eggs to the container of a stand mixer. Beat on medium-high speed for two to three mins till the eggs are light and foamy.
2. Include the sugar, lemon juice, lemon zest, and vanilla. Continue mixing till entirely blended about one min.
3. Put quarter teacup of the egg mixture in a small container and whisk in the cornstarch. Include that back into the container of the stand mixer. Whisk well till fully incorporated.
4. Pour the filling into the cooled crust. Bake for 1eight mins, or till the top is no longer wet.

To make the topping

1. While the filling and crust are baking, in a small saucepan at middling temp., include the sugar, lemon juice, water, and cornstarch. Heat, stirring frequently, till the mixture thickens, two to three mins. Stir in the coconut and take out the pan from the heat.
2. Pour the topping over the baked lemon bars and gently spread it across into an even layer.
3. Chill the pan in the fridge for almost one hr prior to slicing.

Nutrition: Calories: 251; Carbohydrates: 30 gm; Fat: 14 gm; Protein: 3 gm; Fiber: 3 gm; Sodium: 37 mg

286. Flourless Chocolate Cake with Berry Sauce

Preparation Time: twenty mins

Cooking Time: thirty mins

Servings: ten

Ingredients:

For the cake:

- half teacup (or 1 stick) unsalted butter, severed, plus additional for greasing the pan
- 6 oz. dark chocolate, severed
- 2 egg whites
- three-quarter teacup white sugar
- 3 eggs
- half teacup high-quality unsweetened cocoa powder, sifted

For the berry sauce

- two teacups frozen strawberries
- two teacups blueberries
- one-third teacup maple syrup
- two tbsps freshly squeezed lemon juice

Directions:

To make the cake:

1. Warm up the oven to 350 deg.F.
2. Grease the bottom and sides of a nine inch round cake pan with butter. Line the bottom of the pan with parchment paper, and grease the top of the paper with more butter.
3. Using a double boiler or a heatproof container nestled over a pot of boiling water, melt the chocolate and half teacup of butter till smooth, stirring frequently. Take out from the heat and put away.
4. Using an electric mixer, beat the egg whites on medium-high speed till soft peaks form, about three mins. With the mixer running, slowly include the sugar. Mix till just blended.
5. Inside a big container, whisk together the eggs and cocoa powder till just blended.
6. Pour the melted chocolate mixture into the egg mixture and stir to blend. Then, gently fold the egg whites into the batter till just blended, making sure not to overmix. Pour the batter into the cake pan.
7. Bake for around thirty mins, rotating the pan once after fifteen mins. The cake is ready once it's set in the center and begins to pull away from the sides of the pan. Let the cake cool entirely prior to taking it out from the pan.

To make the berry sauce:

1. Put the strawberries, blueberries, maple syrup, and lemon juice in a medium saucepan at medium-high temp. Use the back of a spoon to break down the berries into smaller pieces as they heat. Constantly, stir the sauce till it begins to bubble and thicken, two to three mins.
2. Take out the saucepan from the heat and let the sauce cool prior to serving.

Nutrition: Calories: 296; Carbohydrates: 42 gm; Fat: 16 gm; Protein: 5 gm; Fiber: 4 gm; Sodium: 37 mg

287. Baked Parsnip Chips

Preparation Time: five mins
Cooking Time: thirty mins
Servings: four
Ingredients:

- 3 parsnips
- half tsp extra-virgin olive oil
- A tweak sea salt
- Freshly ground black pepper

Directions:

1. Warm up the oven to 375 deg.F. Line a baking sheet with parchment paper.
2. Using the slicing blade of a food processor (or a mandolin slicer). Thinly slice the parsnips, leaving the skin on.
3. Inside a big container, gently mix the sliced parsnips, olive oil, salt, and pepper, till the slices are coated on both sides.
4. Place the parsnip slices in an even layer on the baking sheet, making sure they don't overlap. Bake for fifteen mins, flip over the chips and bake for fifteen mins more, or till golden brown and crispy.

Nutrition: Calories: 79; Carbohydrates: 18 gm; Fat: 1 gm; Protein: 1 gm; Fiber: 5 gm; Sodium: 49 mg

288. Lemon Ricotta Cake (Crepe Cake Recipe)

Preparation Time: twenty mins
Cooking Time: twenty-five mins
Total time: forty-five mins
Servings: sixteen
Ingredients:

For the ricotta cream filling:

- quarter teacups heavy cream
- half teacup granulated sugar
- one tsp vanilla extract
- 32 oz. ricotta cheese

For the strawberry sauce:

- three teacups fresh strawberries, hulled and divided
- one-third teacup strawberry jam
- Pinch salt
- one teacup Chopped pistachios, optional garnish

For the crepe batter:

- two tbsps melted butter
- two-third teacups whole milk
- quarter teacups water
- two and half teacups all-purpose flour
- three tbsps granulated sugar
- half tsps salt
- 5 big eggs

- 1 lemon zest + one tbsp juice

Directions:

For the ricotta cream filling

1. Inside a blending container, blend the ricotta cheese. Fill a vita-mix blender container halfway with heavy cream, sugar, and vanilla extract. Cover and push the "start" button at level 1. Increase the speed of the machine to level 10 by turning it on. For gentle peaks, blend for 10-15 seconds. Don't over mix, or you'll end up with churned butter!

2. Scoop the whipped cream from the blender jar and mix it gently into the ricotta cheese with a spatula (if you put the ricotta in the blender, it will crumble). Place in the fridge till ready to use.

For the strawberry sauce:

1. Rinse the blender jar well. To the jar, include two teacups cut strawberries, strawberry jam, and a sprinkle of salt: blend and cover. Begin with level 1 and gradually increase the speed till the strawberries are melted. Refrigerate the strawberry sauce in a small jar till ready to serve.

For the crepe batter

1. Rinse the blender jar well. Blend the flour, sugar, salt, eggs, milk, water, melted butter, 1 lemon zest, and one tbsp lemon juice inside a blending container. Cover and mix for 5 seconds on level 1. Then, gradually raise the speed to level 10, till the mixture is foamy. If there are visible flour clumps, scrape the jar's edges. Then, cover and mix for an extra 5-10 seconds.

2. Over medium heat, heat a 9- to 10-inch flat nonstick crepe pan. Once the pan is heated, spoon batter into the center of the crepe pan with a 1/4-cup scoop. Lift and swirl the pan quickly to form a thin 9-inch circle of batter. Return the pan to the stovetop. If you're having problems forming uniform circles, use a spatula to transfer the batter to the pan's sparse spots swiftly.

3. Cook for 30-40 seconds on each side, turning with a broad flat spatula. The first side should have a light golden hue with golden speckles, and the second side should be lighter. Turn the heat up to medium-high if your crepes are taking longer than 90 seconds total per crepe.

4. Repeat with the rest of the crepes on a baking sheet (or plate) coated with parchment paper. The crepes will be brittle, at first, but they will soften in a matter of mins. You should have 20-24 crepes. It is ok to stack them on the sheet. They will not cling together if they are thoroughly cooked.

5. Before proceeding, allow the crepes to cool fully. To expedite the chilling process, place the baking sheet in the fridge.

To assemble:

1. Begin building the cake after the crepes have entirely cooled. One crepe should be placed on a cake stand. Spread quarter teacup ricotta filling in a thin circle over the crepe, leaving a 1/2-inch ring around the edges without cream.

2. Repeat with the rest of the crepes. Spread the ricotta cream and stack crepes till the entire ricotta filling and/or crepes are used. To level out the layers, use a flat plate or baking sheet to push down on the top of the cake.

3. Cover loosely with plastic wrap and keep refrigerated till ready to serve.

To serve:

1. Slice the rest of the one teacup fresh strawberries and put them on top of the cake. Pour some of the strawberry sauce over the strawberries, allowing it to drip down the edges. The leftover sauce should be reserved for pouring over individual slices of cake. If desired, decorate the top of the cake with severed pistachios.

2. When it's time to cut the cake, use a serrated knife to make nice slices with a gently sawing motion. Serve with more strawberry sauce.

Nutrition: Calories: 349; Carbohydrates: 53 gm; Protein: 48 gm; Fat: 2 gm; Cholesterol: 284 mg

289. **Sweet Fried Plantains**

Preparation Time: five mins

Cooking Time: five mins

Total time: ten mins

Servings: six

Ingredients:

- 3 very ripe plantains, yellow with black spots
- 6 tablespoons butter
- Garlic piece smashed
- Salt

Directions:

1. Take out the plantain tips. Skin the plantains and cut them into 12-inch dense ovals, at an angle.

2. Warm up a big sauté pan or cast-iron griddle to medium heat. Then, on the side, place a "holding plate" lined with paper towels.

3. Dissolve the butter in the pan. Once the butter has melted, include the crushed garlic piece and plantain pieces in a single layer to the pan (depending on the size of your pan, you may need to do this in two batches). Fry the plantains till golden brown, around two-three mins on all sides.

4. When the plantains are golden and crisp, transfer them to a holding plate with a slotted spoon. Season generously with salt. If necessary, repeat with the rest of the plantains.

5. Take out the garlic piece. Warm it up with your favorite Mexican or Caribbean dishes!

Notes: Be careful to use plenty of ripe plantains. They should be dark or have big black dots if they are fully ripe. When eaten immediately after being fried, fried plantains offer the finest texture and flavor. However, when they've cooled, you may store leftover plantains in a sealed jar in the fridge for almost three days. Reheat in the oven, toaster, or on the stovetop. I do not advocate freezing fried sweet plantains.

Nutrition: Calories: 210; Carbohydrates: 29 gm; Protein: 17 gm; Fat: 22 gm; Cholesterol: 187 mg

290. <u>French Chocolate Silk Pie Recipe</u>

Preparation Time: thirty mins

Cooking Time: fifteen mins

Total time: forty-five mins

Servings: ten

Ingredients:

- Unbaked pie crust, store-bought or homemade
- 6 oz. bittersweet chocolate + extra for shavings
- half teacups heavy cream
- one teacup unsalted butter softened (2 sticks)
- one teacup granulated sugar, divided
- half tsps vanilla extract
- half tsp salt
- Large pasteurized eggs

Directions:

1. Warm up the oven to 375 deg.F. Fill a big 9-inch pie pan halfway with pie dough. The edges should be crimped. Then, cover the pie shell with parchment paper and fill it with dry beans or ceramic pie weights. Cook for fifteen-twenty mins, or till the edges are golden brown. Allow the pie crust to cool fully after removing the parchment containing the weights.

2. Meanwhile, in a double boiler, melt 6 oz. of chocolate. When the chocolate has melted, take it out from the heat and let it cool to room temp..

3. In the container of an electric mixer, blend the heavy cream and quarter teacup sugar. Whip the cream on high with a whip attachment till it forms firm peaks. Place the whipped cream in a separate dish and put away till ready to use.

4. Using the same mixer container and a paddle attachment, beat the butter and three-quarter teacup sugar on high for almost three mins, or till light and fluffy. Turn the heat to low and gradually include the cooled chocolate to the butter mixture, vanilla, and salt. Scrape down the mixer container and continue to beat till smooth.

5. Increase the speed of the mixer to high. Include 1 egg at a time, allowing the mixer to beat the egg for almost three mins prior to adding the next egg. This results in a super-smooth texture. After 1two mins on high, switch off the mixer. Using a spatula, gently fold in 1/3 of the whipped cream. Fold till the mixture is smooth.

6. Fill the cooled pie shell with the chocolate mixture. Serve with the rest of the whipped cream on top. Then, using a vegetable peeler, shave chocolate over the top. Refrigerate for almost three hrs, or till the chocolate filling has firmed up.

Nutrition: Calories: 549; Carbohydrates: 30 gm; Protein: 54 gm; Fat: 28 gm; Cholesterol: 197 mg

291. <u>Peanut Butter Oatmeal Chocolate Chip Cookies (Monster Cookie Recipe)</u>

Preparation Time: fifteen mins

Cooking Time: fifteen mins

Total time: thirty mins

Servings: fifty-five

Ingredients:

- five and half teacups rolled oats (gluten-free)
- 5 big eggs
- quarter teacup water
- two tbsps vanilla extract
- one teacup unsalted butter, softened (2 sticks)
- three-quarter teacups peanut butter, crunchy or creamy
- half teacups granulated sugar
- half teacups light brown sugar, packed
- half teacup all-purpose flour (or baking flour)
- 4 tablespoons baking powder
- one tsp salt
- 12-oz. semi-sweet chocolate chips
- 12-oz. M&Ms

Directions:

1. Warm up the oven to 350 deg.F. Set aside several baking sheets lined with parchment paper.

2. Measure the oats in a big mixing basin. Then, crack the eggs into the oats; stir in the water and vanilla extract. Allow the liquid to soak the oats prior to stirring to coat.

3. Include the butter to the container of an electric stand mixer. To soften, beat for one min. After that, stir in the peanut butter and both sugars. To break down the sugar crystals, beat on high for three-five mins.

4. Scrape down the sides of the container with a spatula and beat again to incorporate.

5. Mix in the flour, baking powder, and salt with the mixer on low speed. Begin adding the oat mixture, once everything has been thoroughly blended.

6. Scrape the container one more. Then, mix in the chocolate chips on low.

7. Finally, using a spatula, fold the M&Ms into the dough.

8. To distribute the cookie dough onto the prepared baking sheets. Use a big three tbsps of cookie scoop. Place the cookies 2 inches apart on a baking sheet.

9. Bake for fifteen-seventeen mins each batch, or till the edges start to turn golden brown. Cool for three mins on the baking sheets prior to transferring.

Nutrition: Calories: 230; Carbohydrates: 26 gm; Protein: 4 gm; Fat: 7 gm; Cholesterol: 18 mg

Dinner

292. Grilled Pear Cheddar Pockets

Preparation Time: fifteen mins

Cooking time: four mins

Servings: one

Ingredients:

- two tsps Dijon mustard
- half whole grain flatbread
- two slices Cheddar cheese
- quarter teacup arugula
- 1/3 red pear, cored and cut into dense slices

Directions:

1. Spread mustard over the inner side of the flatbread pocket.
2. Place cheese slices and fold them. Then, include pear slices and arugula.
3. Place it into the griddle and cook for three to four mins.

Nutrition: Calories: 223; Fat: 8.6 gm; Carbohydrate: 28.6 gm; Protein: 11.3 gm; Fiber: 6.8 gm

293. Chicken and Apple Kale Wraps

Preparation Time: ten mins

Servings: one

Ingredients:

- one tbsp mayonnaise
- one tsp Dijon mustard
- 3 kale leaves
- 3 oz. chicken breasts, thinly sliced, cooked
- 6 slices red onion, thin
- 1 apple, cut into 9 slices

Directions:

1. Blend the mustard and mayonnaise into the container.
2. Spread onto the kale leaves. Top with one-ounce chicken, three slices of apples, and two slices of onion. Then, roll each kale leaf.
3. Cut in half.

Nutrition: Calories: 370; Fat: 13.7 gm; Carbohydrate: 34.1 gm; Protein: 29.3 gm; Fiber: 6 gm

294. Cauliflower Rice Pilaf

Preparation Time: ten mins

Cooking Time: ten mins

Servings: one

Ingredients:

- six teacups cauliflower florets
- three tbsps extra-virgin olive oil
- 2 garlic pieces, crushed
- half tsp salt
- quarter teacup almonds, toasted, sliced

- quarter teacup herbs, severed
- two tsps lemon zest

Directions:

1. Include cauliflower florets into the food processor and blend till severed.
2. Include oil into the griddle and put it at medium-high flame.
3. Then, include garlic and cook for thirty secs.
4. Include cauliflower rice and season with salt. Let cook for three to five mins.
5. Take out from the flame.
6. Include lemon zest, herbs, and almonds. Stir well.

Nutrition: Calories: 114; Fat: 9.2 gm; Carbohydrate: 6.7 gm; Protein: 3 gm; Fiber: 2.8 gm

295. Fresh Herb and Lemon Bulgur Pilaf

Preparation Time: ten mins

Cooking Time: forty mins

Servings: six

Ingredients:

- two tbsps extra-virgin olive oil
- two teacups onions, severed
- one garlic piece, severed
- one and half teacups bulgur
- half tsp ground turmeric
- half tsp ground cumin
- two teacups vegetable or chicken broth, low-sodium
- one and half teacups carrot, severed
- two tsps fresh ginger, grated or severed
- one tsp salt
- quarter teacup fresh dill, severed
- quarter teacup fresh mint, severed
- quarter teacup parsley, severed
- three tbsps lemon juice
- half teacup walnuts, severed, toasted

Directions:

1. Include oil into the griddle and put it at medium flame.
2. Include onion and cook for twelve to eighteen mins.
3. Include garlic and cook for one min.
4. Then, include cumin, turmeric, and bulgur. Cook for one min.
5. Include salt, ginger, carrot, and broth. Bring it to a boil over medium-high flame, about fifteen mins.
6. Take out from the flame.
7. Let rest for five mins.
8. Include lemon juice, parsley, dill, and mint into the pilaf. Stir well.
9. Garnish with walnuts.

Nutrition: Calories: 273; Fat: 11.7 gm; Carbohydrate: 38.8 gm; Protein: 7.3 gm; Fiber: 7.7 gm

296. Corn Chowder

Preparation Time: ten mins

Cooking Time: five hrs

Servings: six

Ingredients:

- three-quarter teacup yellow split peas, split
- 28 oz. chicken broth, low-sodium
- one teacup water
- 12 oz. corn kernels, frozen
- half teacup red sweet peppers, severed and roasted
- 4 oz. green chilies, cubed
- one tsp ground cumin
- half tsp dried oregano, crushed
- half tsp dried thyme, crushed
- half teacup cream cheese

Directions:

1. Rinse split peas underwater.
2. Mix the thyme, oregano, cumin, chilies, red peppers, corn, water, split peas, and chicken broth and cook on high heat for five to six hours.
3. Let it cool for ten mins.
4. Transfer two cups of soup into the food processor and blend till smooth.
5. Include pureed soup into the slow cooker. Then, include cream cheese and whisk to blend. Cook for five mins.
6. Serve!

Nutrition: Calories: 222; Fat: 7.5 gm; Carbohydrate: 29.8 gm; Protein: 10.5 gm; Fiber: 7.7 gm

297. Strawberry and Rhubarb Soup

Preparation Time: five mins

Cooking Time: thirty mins

Servings: four

Ingredients:

- four teacups rhubarb
- three teacups water
- one and half teacups strawberries, sliced
- quarter teacup sugar
- one-eighth tsp salt
- one-third teacup mint or basil, severed
- Ground pepper, as required

Directions:

1. Include three cups of water and rhubarb into the saucepan.
2. Cook for five mins till softened.
3. Transfer it to the container.

4. Include 2-inch ice water into the container and keep it aside with rhubarb.
5. Place it into the fridge for twenty mins.
6. Transfer the rhubarb to the blender. Then, include salt, sugar, and strawberries and blend till smooth.
7. Place it back in the container. Include basil or mint.
8. Serve!

Nutrition: Calories: 95; Fat: 0.5 gm; Carbohydrate: 23.1 gm; Protein: 1.6 gm; Fiber: 3.5 gm

298. Chicken Sandwiches

Preparation Time: five mins

Cooking Time: thirty mins

Servings: four

Ingredients:

- 4 slices red onion
- 1 red sweet pepper, seeded and quartered
- 6 oz. Chicken breasts, boneless, cut in half, horizontally
- 4 multi-grain sandwich round, split
- two tbsps basil pesto
- two tbsps Kalamata olives, pitted and severed
- one-third teacup Mozzarella cheese, shredded
- quarter teacup Feta cheese, low-fat, crumbled

Directions:

1. Heat the griddle over medium flame.
2. Let coat with pepper and red onion with non-stick cooking spray.
3. Include it to the pan and cook for six to eight mins.
4. Take out from the griddle. Let coat the chicken with non-stick cooking spray.
5. Include chicken to the grill pan and cook for three to five mins.
6. Take out from the griddle.
7. Pull chicken into shreds. Cut pepper into strips.
8. To assemble the sandwiches: Spread the pesto onto the sandwich and sprinkle with olives. Place grilled onion slices. Top with pepper strips.
9. Place chicken over it. Spray with feta cheese and mozzarella cheese.
10. Then, place griddle over medium-low flame.
11. Place the sandwich into the griddle and cook for three to four mins.
12. Flip and cook for three to four mins.
13. Serve!

Nutrition: Calories: 296; Fat: 10 gm; Carbohydrate: 27.7 gm; Protein: 25.8 gm; Fiber: 6.2 gm

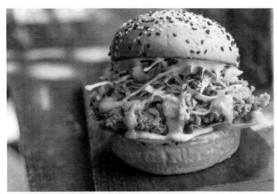

299. Tex-Mex Bean Tostadas

Preparation Time: ten mins

Cooking Time: fifteen mins

Servings: four

Ingredients:

- 4 tostada shells
- 16 oz. Pinto beans, rinsed and drained
- half teacup salsa, prepared
- half tsp chipotle seasoning
- half teacup Cheddar cheese, shredded
- one and half teacups Iceberg lettuce
- one teacup tomato, severed
- 1 lime wedges

Instruction:

1. Warm up the oven to 350 deg.F.
2. Place tostada shells onto the baking sheet. Bake for three to five mins.
3. Meanwhile, mix the seasoning, salsa, and bean into the container.
4. Mash the mixture with a potato masher.
5. Then, divide the bean mixture between tostada shells.
6. Top with half of the cheese. Bake for five mins.
7. Top with severed tomato and shredded lettuce.
8. Then, place the rest of the cheese and lime wedges.

Nutrition: Calories: 230; Fat: 6 gm; Carbohydrate: 33 gm; Protein: 12 gm; Fiber: 6 gm

300. Fish Tacos

Preparation Time: ten mins

Cooking Time: fifteen mins

Servings: four

Ingredients:

- one lb. tilapia fillets
- two tsps extra-virgin olive oil
- two tsps chipotle seasoning blend
- two teacups coleslaw mix
- two tbsps salad dressing Ranch
- 8 whole wheat tortillas
- ½ avocado, thinly sliced

- quarter teacup cilantro leaves
- 1 lime, quartered

Directions:

1. Warm up the oven to 450 deg.F.
2. Place fillets onto the baking dish and brush the fish with oil.
3. Spray with seasoning.
4. Bake for four to six mins.
5. Meanwhile, mix the dressing and coleslaw into a container. Put it away.
6. Flake the fish into big chunks and place them into the tortillas.
7. Top with lime, cilantro, avocado, and coleslaw mixture.

Nutrition: Calories: 341; Fat: 12 gm; Carbohydrate: 30.5 gm; Protein: 29.5 gm; Fiber: 21.2 gm

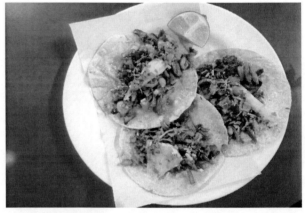

301. Cucumber Almond Gazpacho

Preparation Time: twenty mins

Chill time: two hrs

Servings: five

Ingredients:

- two English cucumbers
- two teacups yellow bell pepper, severed
- two teacups whole wheat bread
- one and half teacups unsweetened almond milk
- half teacup almonds, toasted, slivered
- 5 teaspoons olive oil
- two tsps white-wine vinegar
- one garlic piece
- half tsp salt

Directions:

1. Dice unskinned cucumber and mix with half a cup bell pepper.
2. Peel the rest of the cucumbers and cut them into chunks.
3. Include rest of the bell pepper, skinned cucumber, salt, garlic, vinegar, oil, six tablespoons of almonds,

almond milk, and bread into the blender. Blend till smooth. Let chill for two hours.

4. Garnish with the rest of the two tbsps of almonds.
5. Spray with oil.

Nutrition: Calories: 201; Fat: 11.8 gm; Carbohydrate: 19 gm; Protein: 6.3 gm; Fiber: 4.3 gm

302. Pea and Spinach Carbonara

Preparation Time: five mins

Cooking Time: fifteen mins

Servings: four

Ingredients:

- 1 ½ tablespoon extra-virgin olive oil
- half teacup Panko breadcrumbs (whole-wheat)
- 1 garlic piece, crushed
- eight tbsps Parmesan cheese, grated
- three tbsps fresh parsley, severed
- 3 egg yolks
- 1 egg
- half tsp ground pepper
- quarter tsp salt
- 9 oz. Tagliatelle or Linguine
- eight teacups baby spinach
- one teacup peas

Directions:

1. Include ten cups of water into the pot and boil it over high flame.
2. During this, include oil into the griddle and cook at medium-high flame.
3. Include garlic and breadcrumbs. Cook for two mins till toasted.
4. Transfer it to the small container. Include parsley and two tablespoons of Parmesan cheese. Put it away.
5. Whisk the salt, pepper, egg, egg yolks, and six tablespoons of Parmesan cheese into the container.
6. Include pasta to the boiling water; cook it for one min.
7. Include spinach and peas; cook for one min more till tender.
8. Save quarter teacup of the cooking water for your next use. Drain it and place it into the container.
9. Whisk the reserved cooking water into the egg mixture, include it to the pasta. Toss to blend.
10. Top with breadcrumb mixture and serve!

Nutrition: Calories: 430; Carbohydrates: 54.1 gm; Protein: 20.2 gm; Fat: 14.5 gm; Fiber: 8.2 gm

303. Sautéed Broccoli with Peanut Sauce

Preparation Time: five mins

Cooking Time: ten mins

Servings: six

Ingredients:

- eight teacups broccoli florets

- two tbsps sesame oil, toasted
- one teacup red bell pepper, sliced
- half teacup yellow onion, sliced
- three garlic pieces, severed
- three tbsps peanut butter
- 2 ½ tablespoons tamari, low-sodium
- two tbsps rice vinegar
- one tbsp brown sugar
- one tsp cornstarch
- one tbsp sesame seeds, toasted

Directions:

1. Include water into the pot and boil it. Then, include broccoli and cook for three to four mins till tender.
2. During this, include oil into the griddle; cook at medium-high flame.
3. Include garlic, onion, and bell pepper. Cook for three mins.
4. Include steamed broccoli and cook for three mins. Stir well.
5. Whisk the cornstarch, sugar, vinegar, tamari, and peanut butter into the container. Include vegetables and stir well.
6. Let cook for one min. Top with sesame seeds.
7. Serve and relish!

Nutrition: Calories: 154; Carbohydrates: 12 gm; Protein: 6 gm; Fat: 9.7 gm; Fiber: 3.4 gm

304. Edamame Lettuce Wraps Burgers

Preparation Time: five mins

Cooking Time: twenty-five mins

Servings: four

Ingredients:

- one teacup carrots, julienned
- three tbsps lime juice
- two tsps chili-garlic sauce
- one and half teacups shelled edamame, thawed
- one teacup cooked brown rice
- half teacup peanut butter powder
- quarter teacup scallions, severed
- one tbsp Red Thai curry paste
- three tbsps peanut oil
- two tbsps Tamari, low-sodium
- 4 leaves Bibb lettuce
- one teacup red onion, thinly sliced

Directions:

1. Firstly, toss carrots with one teaspoon chili garlic sauce and two tablespoons of lime juice. Put it away.

2. Include tamari, one tablespoon oil, curry paste, scallions, edamame rice, and quarter teacup peanut butter powder into the blender. Blend till smooth.

3. Shape the mixture into four burgers.

4. Include two tablespoons of oil into the griddle and cook at medium flame.

5. Include burgers and cook for three to four mins on all sides.

6. When done, transfer them to the plate.

7. During this, whisk the one teaspoon chili garlic sauce, tamari, one tablespoon lime juice, and quarter teacup peanut butter powder into the container till smooth.

8. Then, drain the carrots. Include marinade to the peanut sauce. Stir well.

9. Wrap burger in lettuce leaves and top with sauce, onions, and carrots.

Nutrition: Calories: 310; Carbohydrates: 31.6 gm; Protein: 14.6 gm; Fat: 14.5 gm; Fiber: 7.6 gm

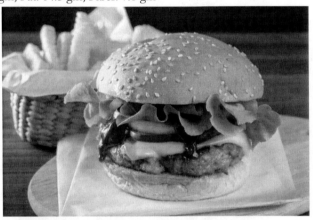

305. Pizza Stuffed Spaghetti Squash

Preparation Time: ten mins

Cooking Time: one hr

Servings: four

Ingredients:

- 3 pounds spaghetti squash, halved lengthwise and seeded
- quarter teacup water
- two tbsps extra-virgin olive oil
- one teacup onion, severed
- two garlic pieces, crushed
- 8 oz. mushrooms, sliced
- one teacup bell pepper, severed
- two teacups no-salt-added crushed tomatoes
- one tsp Italian seasoning
- half tsp ground pepper
- quarter tsp crushed red pepper, crushed
- quarter tsp salt
- 2 oz. pepperoni, halved
- one teacup part-skim Mozzarella cheese, shredded

- two tbsps Parmesan cheese, grated

Directions:

1. Warm up the oven to 450 deg.F.

2. Include squash into the microwave-safe dish. Then, include water.

3. Let microwave it for ten to twelve mins till tender.

4. Then, place it into the oven and bake for forty to fifty mins at 400 deg.F.

5. During this, include oil into the griddle; cook at medium flame.

6. Include garlic and onion. Cook for three to four mins.

7. Include bell pepper and mushrooms. Cook for five mins more till tender.

8. Include salt, crushed red pepper, pepper, Italian seasoning, and tomatoes. Cook for two mins.

9. When done, take out from the flame.

10. Include ten to twelve pepperoni halves and cover them with a lid.

11. Scrape the squash from the shells and place it into the container.

12. Include salt, pepper, mozzarella, and Parmesan cheese. Stir well.

13. Include tomato mixture to the container. Stir well.

14. Place squash shells onto the rimmed baking sheet and divide the filling among the halves; top with pepperoni and mozzarella cheese. Put it into the oven and bake for fifteen mins.

15. Let broil it for one to two mins.

16. Serve and relish!

Nutrition: Calories: 373; Carbohydrates: 32.2 gm; Protein: 16.4 gm; Fat: 20.6 gm; Fiber: 7.5 gm

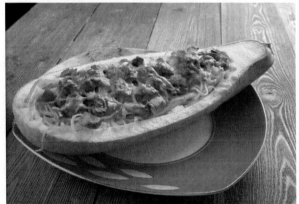

306. Spinach and Artichoke Dip Pasta

Preparation Time: five mins

Cooking Time: fifteen mins

Servings: four

Ingredients:

- 8 oz. whole-wheat Rotini
- 5 oz. baby spinach, severed
- 4 oz. cream cheese, low-fat, cut into chunks

- three-quarter teacup milk, low-fat
- half teacup parmesan cheese, grated
- two tsps garlic powder
- quarter tsp ground pepper
- 14 oz. artichoke hearts, rinsed, squeezed dry and severed

Directions:

1. Include water into the saucepan and boil it. Include pasta and cook it. Then, drain it.
2. Mix the one tablespoon water and spinach into the saucepan. Cook over medium flame. Cook for two mins till wilted.
3. Transfer it to the container. Include milk and cream to the pan and whisk it well.
4. Include pepper, garlic powder, and parmesan cheese and cook till thickened. Drain spinach and include to the sauce with pasta and artichoke. Cook it well.
5. Then, serve and relish!

Nutrition: Calories: 371; Carbohydrates: 56.1 gm; Protein: 16.6 gm; Fat: 9.1 gm; Fiber: 7.9 gm

307. Grilled Eggplant

Preparation Time: five mins
Cooking Time: forty mins
Servings: four
Ingredients:

- four teacups water
- one teacup cornmeal
- one tbsp butter
- half tsp salt
- one lb. plum tomatoes, severed
- 4 tablespoons extra-virgin olive oil
- two tsps fresh oregano, severed
- 1 garlic piece, grated
- half tsp ground pepper
- quarter tsp crushed red pepper
- one and half lbs. eggplant, cut into half-inch-dense slices
- quarter teacup Feta cheese, crumbled
- half teacup fresh basil, severed

Directions:

1. Include water into the saucepan and boil it over high flame.
2. Include cornmeal and whisk it well. Then, lower the heat and cook for thirty-five mins till tender.
3. When done, take out from the flame. Include salt and butter. Stir well.
4. During this, preheat the grill at medium-high temp.
5. Include salt, crushed red pepper, pepper, garlic, oregano, three tablespoons oil, and tomatoes into the container; toss to blend.

6. Rub eggplant with one tablespoon oil and place onto the grill. Cook for four mins on all sides. Let it cool for ten mins.
7. Chop it and include to the tomatoes.
8. Spray with fresh basil leaves.
9. Place vegetable mixture over the polenta and top with cheese.

Nutrition: Calories: 354; Carbohydrates: 39 gm; Protein: 6.8 gm; Fat: 20.6 gm; Fiber: 8.4 gm

308. Stuffed Potatoes with Salsa and Beans

Preparation Time: five mins
Cooking Time: twenty mins
Servings: four
Ingredients:

- 4 russet potatoes
- half teacup fresh salsa
- 1 avocado, sliced
- 15 oz. Pinto beans, rinsed, warmed, and mashed
- 4 teaspoons Jalapeños, severed, and pickled

Directions:

1. Firstly, pierce potatoes using a fork.
2. Let microwave for twenty mins at middling temp..
3. Place onto the cutting board and let it cool.
4. Cut to open the potato lengthwise and tweak the ends to expose the flesh. Top with Jalapeño, beans, avocado, and salsa.
5. Serve and relish!

Nutrition: Calories: 324; Carbohydrates: 56.7 gm; Protein: 9.2 gm; Fat: 8 gm; Fiber: 11 gm

309. Mushroom Quinoa Veggie Burgers

Preparation Time: five mins
Cooking Time: twenty-five mins
Chill time: one hr
Servings: four
Ingredients:

- 1 Portobello mushroom, gills taken out, and severed
- one teacup black beans, rinsed, and unsalted
- two tbsps almond butter, creamy and unsalted
- three tbsps canola mayonnaise
- one tsp ground pepper
- ¾ teaspoon smoked paprika
- ¾ teaspoon garlic powder
- half tsp salt
- half teacup cooked quinoa
- quarter teacup old-fashioned rolled oats
- one tbsp Ketchup
- one tsp Dijon mustard
- one tbsp extra-virgin olive oil

- 4 whole-wheat hamburger buns, toasted
- 2 green lettuce leaves, halved
- 4 tomatoes, sliced
- 4 red onions, thinly sliced

Directions:

1. Include salt, half teaspoon garlic powder, paprika, pepper, one tablespoon mayonnaise, almond butter, black beans, and mushrooms into the food processor. Blend till smooth.
2. Transfer it to the container. Include oats and quinoa; stir well.
3. Place it into the fridge for one hour.
4. During this, whisk the quarter tsp garlic powder, two tablespoons mayonnaise, mustard, and ketchup into the container till smooth.
5. Make the mixture into four patties.
6. Include oil into the non-stick griddle and cook at medium-high flame.
7. Fry patties for four to five mins.
8. Flip and cook for two to four mins till golden brown.
9. Top burger with onion, tomato, lettuce, and sauce.

Nutrition: Calories: 395; Carbohydrates: 45.9 gm; Protein: 11.6 gm; Fat: 19.8 gm; Fiber: 9.4 gm

310. **Turkey Meatballs**

Preparation Time: fifteen mins

Cooking Time: twenty-five mins

Servings: four

Ingredients:

- one tsp olive oil
- three teacups button mushrooms, sliced
- 1 egg, beaten
- one-third teacup quick-cooking rolled oats
- one-third teacup Parmesan cheese, grated
- 3 garlic pieces, crushed
- two tsps dried Italian seasoning, crushed
- half tsp salt
- quarter tsp ground pepper
- 1 ¼ lb. lean ground turkey

Directions:

1. Warm up the oven to 400 deg.F.
2. Line a baking pan with foil; coat it with cooking spray.
3. Include oil into the griddle and cook at medium flame.
4. Include mushroom and cook for eight to ten mins.
5. Transfer it to the blender. Blend till severed.
6. Mix the pepper, salt, Italian seasoning, garlic, parmesan cheese, oats, and egg into the container. Include severed mushrooms and turkey. Blend well.
7. Place meat mixture onto the cutting board and cut into thirty squared.

8. Roll each square into the ball and place it onto the pan. Bake for twelve to fifteen mins.
9. Serve and relish!

Nutrition: Calories: 467; Carbohydrates: 49.2 gm; Protein: 36.3 gm; Fat: 16.1 gm; Fiber: 7.6 gm

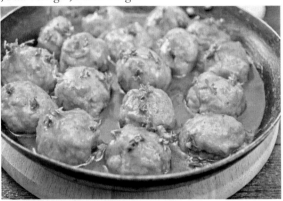

311. **Sweet Potato Soup**

Preparation Time: fifteen mins

Cooking Time: thirty mins

Servings: six

Ingredients:

- quarter teacup canola oil
- 4 corn tortillas, halved and thinly sliced
- ¾ teaspoon salt
- 1 Poblano pepper, seeded and severed
- one onion, severed
- two tbsps chili powder
- four teacups chicken broth or vegetable broth
- one and half lbs. sweet potatoes, skinned and cut into half-inch pieces
- 14 oz. tomatoes, unsalted, pitted, and cubed
- 15 oz. black beans, low-sodium, rinsed
- three tbsps lime juice
- 3 radishes, halved and thinly sliced
- quarter teacup pumpkin seeds, roasted, and unsalted
- half teacup Queso Fresco, crumbled
- 1 avocado, severed

Directions:

1. Include oil into the pot and cook at medium flame.
2. Include tortilla strips. Cook for five mins till crispy.
3. Transfer it to the plate, lined with a paper towel. Use a slotted spoon.
4. Spray with quarter tsp salt.
5. Include half teaspoon salt, chili powder, onion, and poblano. Cook for two mins till softened.
6. Include tomatoes, beans, broth, and sweet potatoes; simmer for twenty mins.

7. Include lime juice into the soup; top with tortilla strips, avocado, queso fresco, pepitas, and radish slices. Stir well.

8. Serve and relish!

Nutrition: Calories: 412; Carbohydrates: 45 gm; Protein: 13.5 gm; Fat: 21.6 gm; Fiber: 11.7 gm

312. Minestrone Soup

Preparation Time: five mins

Cooking Time: twenty-five mins

Servings: six

Ingredients:

- 5 garlic pieces, crushed
- three tbsps extra-virgin olive oil
- one teacup whole-grain rustic bread, cubed
- one teacup leek, severed, white and light green parts only
- one teacup carrot, severed
- three teacups vegetable broth
- three teacups water
- ¾ teaspoon Kosher salt
- one teacup Ditalini pasta
- 10 oz. Zucchini, halved lengthwise and thinly sliced
- 15 oz. Cannellini beans, unsalted, rinsed
- three teacups Kale, severed
- one teacup frozen peas, thawed
- ½ ground pepper

Directions:

1. Warm up the oven to 350 deg.F.
2. Include two tbsps of oil and garlic. Cook over medium flame for three to four mins.
3. Include bread and toss to blend. Place mixture onto the baking sheet and bake for eight to ten mins.
4. During this, include one tablespoon oil into the pot; cook at medium-high flame. Include carrots and leek. Cook for five to six mins.
5. Include salt, water, and broth. Cover with a lid and boil it over a high flame. Include pasta and lower the heat to medium-high. Cook for five mins. Include zucchini and cook for five mins till al dente.
6. Include pepper, peas, kale, and beans. Stir well. Let cook for two mins.
7. Place soup into the six bowls. Top with croutons.

Nutrition: Calories: 267; Carbohydrates: 38.7 gm; Protein: 9.7 gm; Fat: 8.6 gm; Fiber: 7.2 gm

313. Lentil Soup

Preparation Time: five mins

Cooking Time: one hr

Servings: six

Ingredients

- one onion, severed
- quarter teacup olive oil
- two carrots, cubed
- two celery stalks, severed
- 2 garlic pieces, crushed
- one tsp dried oregano
- one bay leaf
- one tsp dried basil
- 14.5 oz. crushed tomatoes
- two teacups dry lentils
- eight teacups water
- half teacup spinach, rinsed and thinly sliced
- two tbsps vinegar
- Salt and ground black pepper, as required

Directions:

1. Include oil into the pot and cook at medium flame.
2. Include celery, carrots, and onions. Cook till tender.
3. Include basil, oregano, bay leaf, garlic; stir well and cook for two mins.
4. Include tomatoes, water, and lentils. Stir well. Let it boil.
5. Lower the heat and simmer for one hour.
6. Include spinach and cook till wilted.
7. Include pepper, salt, and vinegar. Stir well.

Nutrition: Calories: 349; Carbohydrates: 48.2 gm; Protein: 18.3 gm; Fat: 10 gm; Fiber: 22.1 gm

314. Grilled Corn Salad

Preparation Time: fifteen mins

Cooking Time: ten mins

Additional time: forty-five mins

Servings: six

Ingredients:

- 6 ears freshly shucked corn
- 1 green pepper, cubed
- 2 plum tomatoes, cubed
- quarter teacup red onion, cubed
- ½ bunch fresh cilantro, severed
- two tsps olive oil
- Salt and ground black pepper, as required

Directions:

1. Warm up the grill at middling temp. Oil the grate.
2. Place corn onto the grill and cook for ten mins. Put it away.
3. Let cool it. Cut the kernels off the cob and place them into the medium container.
4. Mix the olive oil, cilantro, onion, cubed tomato, green pepper, and corn kernels; sprinkle with pepper and salt.
5. Toss to blend. Let stand for thirty mins.

6. Serve and relish!

Nutrition: Calories: 103; Carbohydrates: 19.7 gm; Protein: 3.4 gm; Fat: 2.8 gm; Fiber: 3.3 gm

315. Kale Soup

Preparation Time: twenty-five mins

Cooking Time: thirty mins

Servings: eight

Ingredients:

- two tbsps olive oil
- one yellow onion, severed
- two tbsps garlic
- one bunch kale, stems taken out, and leaves severed
- six teacups water
- six cubes vegetable bouillon
- 15 oz. tomatoes, cubed
- six white potatoes, skinned and cubed
- 30 oz. Cannellini beans, drained
- one tbsp Italian seasoning
- two tbsps dried parsley
- Salt and pepper, as required

Directions:

1. Include olive oil into the pot and heat it.
2. Include garlic and onion. Cook till softened.
3. Include kale and stir; cook for two mins.
4. Include parsley, Italian seasoning, beans, potatoes, tomatoes, vegetable bouillon, and water. Stir well. Let simmer for twenty-five mins.
5. Spray with pepper and salt.

Nutrition: Calories: 277; Carbohydrates: 50.9 gm; Protein: 9.6 gm; Fat: 4.5 gm; Fiber: 10.3 gm

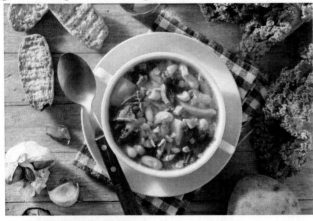

316. Pasta Fagioli

Preparation Time: ten mins

Cooking Time: thirty mins

Servings: four

Ingredients:

- one tbsp olive oil
- one carrot
- 1 celery stalk, cubed
- 1 onion, cubed, thinly sliced
- ½ garlic, severed
- 8 oz. tomato sauce
- 14 oz. chicken broth
- Ground black pepper, as required
- one tbsp dried parsley
- ½ dried basil leaves
- fifteen oz. cannellini beans, drained and rinsed
- one and half teacups Ditalini pasta

Directions:

1. Include olive oil into the saucepan and heat it over medium flame.
2. Include onion, celery, and carrot. Cook till fragrant.
3. Include garlic and cook it well. Include basil, parsley, pepper, chicken broth, and tomato sauce; simmer for twenty mins.
4. Include salt and water into the pot and boil. Include Ditalini pasta and cook for eight mins till al dente. Let it drain.
5. Include beans to the sauce mixture. Simmer for a couple of mins.
6. When pasta is done, include bean mixture and sauce. Stir well.
7. Serve and relish!

Nutrition: Calories: 338; Carbohydrates: 60.7 gm; Protein: 13.4 gm; Fat: 5.1 gm; Fiber: 9.4 gm

317. Sweet Potato Gnocchi

Preparation Time: thirty mins

Cooking Time: thirty-five mins

Servings: four

Ingredients:

- 8 oz. sweet potatoes
- 1 garlic piece, pressed
- half tsp salt
- half tsp ground nutmeg
- one egg
- two teacups all-purpose flour

Directions:

1. Warm up the oven to 350 deg.F.
2. Let the potatoes bake for thirty mins till softened.
3. When done, take them out from the oven and let them cool.
4. When cooled, peel and mash the potatoes; include them to the container.
5. Include egg, nutmeg, salt, and garlic and mix well.
6. Include flour and blend well.
7. Include water and salt into the pot and boil it.

8. To prepare the gnocchi: Roll the dough onto the floured surface and cut it into sections.

9. Include pieces into the boiled water; cook till they floated on the surface.

10. When done, take out and serve!

11. Top with cream sauce or butter.

Nutrition: Calories: 346; Carbohydrates: 71.1 gm; Protein: 9.9 gm; Fat: 2.1 gm; Fiber: 5.2 gm

318. Bean and Ham Soup

Preparation Time: twenty-five mins

Cooking Time: ten hrs

Servings: twelve

Ingredients:

- 2 sweet potatoes
- one garlic piece, pressed
- half tsp salt
- half tsp ground nutmeg
- 1 egg
- two teacups all-purpose flour
- 20 oz. bean mixture, soaked overnight
- 1 ham bone
- two and half teacups ham, cubed
- 1 onion, severed
- 3 stalks celery, severed
- 5 carrots, severed
- 14.5 oz. tomatoes, cubed, with liquid
- 12 fluid oz. vegetable juice, low-sodium
- three teacups vegetable broth
- two tbsps Worcestershire sauce
- two tbsps Dijon mustard
- one tbsp chili powder
- 3 bay leaves
- one tsp ground black pepper
- one tbsp dried parsley
- three tbsps lemon
- 7 cups chicken broth, low-sodium
- one tsp Kosher salt

Directions:

1. Include soaked beans into the pot, and then include water till it covers the beans. Let boil it on low flame for thirty mins. Then, drain it.

2. Include vegetable broth, vegetable juice, tomatoes, carrots, celery, onion, ham, and ham bone. Spray with lemon juice, parsley, pepper, bay leaf, chili powder, Dijon mustard, and Worcestershire sauce.

3. Include chicken broth. Simmer on low flame for eight hours.

4. Include more chicken broth as required. Take out the ham bone. Spray with salt.

5. Let simmer for two hours more.

6. Discard bay leaves.

Nutrition: Calories: 260; Carbohydrates: 37.9 gm; Protein: 17.3 gm; Fat: 3.6 gm; Fiber: 14.8 gm

Conclusion

Diverticulitis is a digestive disease that can strike anyone at any point in their lifetime, but it's most common in older people.

If a person has severe diverticulitis symptoms, the doctor may recommend a liquid diverticulitis diet, which includes water, fruit juices, broth, and ice pops as part of the treatment. Then, you can gradually return to a regular diet. Before introducing high-fiber foods, the doctor may recommend you to start with low-fiber foods like white meat, white bread, poultry, fish, eggs, and dairy products. Fiber softens and bulks up stools, allowing them to pass through the colon more easily. It also helps to relieve pressure in the intestines. According to numerous studies, diverticular symptoms can be controlled by eating fiber-rich foods.

Women under the age of 51 should ingest 25 grams of fiber per day. Pasta, whole-grain bread, cereals, kidney and black beans, fresh fruits like apples, pears, prunes, and vegetables like squash, potatoes, peas, spinach, and other vegetables are high in fiber. Therefore, ensure these foods should be included in your diet to help you overcome Diverticulitis.

A high-fiber, high-water diet is usually recommended for diverticulitis. It will ensure that your gastrointestinal tract and system get enough rest, allowing you to recuperate. As soon as you start eating properly, you should see results in a few days.

Water intake is equally important: the usual guideline is that your body will need 1/2 of your weight in oz. per day so that a 150-pound person will require 75 oz. of water each day. Water coupled with a high fiber diet is required to keep your colon moving properly and reduce the risk of an attack or the formation of further diverticula.

If your diverticulitis diet plan allows it, try to consume fruits and vegetables that you like. If you don't like greens, consider eating more fresh fruit instead, and vice versa. Vegetable and fruit seeds are safe to eat for most patients, such as those found in cucumbers and tomatoes.

Foods that are high in fiber. Whole-wheat bread and other whole-grain items are high in dietary fiber. You may also include bran to your food. Uncooked or just lightly cooked legumes, as well as fermented greens (e.g., sauerkraut). Fresh fruit and vegetables should not be skinned: they should be consumed naturally (juices are devoid of fiber). Dried fruit, such as raisins, plums, apricots, and dates, are an excellent source.

Naturally, just as we don't all consume the same kind of meals throughout life, diverticulitis foods to avoid will vary from case to instance. Our unhealthy eating habits and poor nutrition and the poisons that arise from them are the root reasons. It's an excellent time to become interested in health and nutrition if you haven't already guessed.

If you wish to reduce or perhaps eliminate future episodes of diverticulitis, you need to eat the right foods. While antibiotics may frequently alleviate severe pain and suffering in the short term, taking them for an extended length of time can be nearly as hazardous as the illness itself, not to mention that your body will ultimately become resistant to their effects.

Consequently, it is often essential to undergo a hazardous and invasive operation, which may result in a decrease in life quality.

Most people would agree that prevention is preferable to treatment. So, to avoid this illness from infecting your stomach, and in light of the current economic climate, we should pay close attention to our health and take appropriate action. Because it is nearly entirely due to a lack of dietary fiber, the best course of treatment is to consume the appropriate meals.

Made in United States
North Haven, CT
22 November 2023

44403968R00065